BEAUTY AND FITNESS: A HOLISTIC GUIDE TO HEALTH AND WELLNESS

Achieve Inner and Outer Radiance through Health, Mindfulness, and Strength

Veronica Balthazar

CONTENTS

DISCLAIMER

The content on "Beauty & Fitness: A Holistic Approach to Wellness" is for informational purposes only and is not intended to be a substitute for professional medical advice, diagnosis, or treatment. Always seek the advice of your physician or other qualified health provider with any questions you may have regarding a medical condition or fitness regimen.

The author and publisher assume no responsibility for any injury, loss or damage that may result from following the advice, routines or information contained in this book. Before beginning any exercise, fitness or diet program, it is recommended that you consult a healthcare professional, especially if you have any pre-existing health conditions or concerns.

Individual results may vary. This book is intended to guide you toward achieving your personal wellness goals, but success depends on a variety of factors, including individual effort and consistency.

INTRODUCTION: BEAUTY AND FITNESS: A HOLISTIC GUIDE TO HEALTH AND WELLNESS

Beauty and fitness are two essential components that form the foundation of a healthy, fulfilling lifestyle. Although beauty and fitness may seem like separate disciplines, they are deeply intertwined, each contributing to our overall well-being in unique ways. The pursuit of outer beauty often leads to inner well-being, and efforts to improve physical fitness lead to a more youthful, radiant appearance. This book explores the holistic relationship between beauty and fitness, offering you practical insights and strategies to enhance both at once.

In today's world, the definition of beauty has evolved beyond makeup and skincare. True beauty stems from a combination of mental, physical, and emotional wellness, all of which are influenced by our daily habits and routines. Similarly, fitness is no longer just about maintaining a fit figure. Fitness is about strength, stamina, flexibility, and mental endurance. Together, beauty and fitness create a harmonious balance that can elevate every aspect of your life.

THE IMPORTANCE OF A COMPREHENSIVE APPROACH

Beauty and fitness are two sides of the same coin, and to achieve the best results, we must take a holistic approach. This means taking care of our bodies from the inside out. Healthy skin, shiny hair, and a radiant glow are external reflections of our inner health. When we nourish ourselves with the right foods, follow an effective exercise routine, and maintain positive mental health, we not only feel good, but we also look our best.

This book is divided into four parts, each focusing on different aspects of beauty and fitness:

- **Beauty Basics** : This section will cover skincare routines, anti-aging tips, makeup techniques, hair care, and more, giving you the tools to enhance your natural beauty.
- **Fitness Basics** : Focusing on different types of exercise, from strength training to cardio, we'll explore how fitness can improve your physical health and appearance.
- **Nutrition for Beauty and Fitness** : What we eat has a profound impact on how we look and feel. This section will highlight foods that promote healthy skin, hair, and body composition, as well as meal planning tips.
- **Mind-Body Connection** : Beauty and fitness are also influenced by our mental and emotional health. We will explore the role of mindfulness, stress management, and sleep in maintaining beauty and fitness.

WHY BEAUTY AND FITNESS MATTER

For centuries, humans have been drawn to beauty, but it's not just a superficial desire. Beauty, in the context of self-care and health, is an indicator of overall well-being. When we take care of our skin, hair, and body, we not only improve our appearance, but also our self-confidence and mental health. Physical fitness, on the other hand, is vital to maintaining strength, flexibility, and mental clarity. A healthy body and fitness translate into increased energy levels, improved posture, and improved stamina, all of which contribute to a positive self-image.

In today's fast-paced world, it's easy to neglect self-care, but it's more important than ever. Beauty and fitness routines provide a sense of control and routine in our often chaotic lives. They provide an opportunity to reconnect with ourselves, focus on our well-being, and cultivate self-love. By adopting a balanced approach to beauty and fitness, you can transform not only your appearance but also your mindset and overall quality of life.

WHAT TO EXPECT IN THIS BOOK

In this book's chapters, you'll find a mix of practical advice, science-backed information, and practical tips that you can incorporate into your daily routine. Whether you're looking to revamp your skincare routine, start a fitness journey, or improve your diet, you'll discover a wealth of knowledge to guide you every step of the way.

Each chapter delves into specific topics in depth, such as:

- How to create an effective morning and evening skincare routine.
- The best anti-aging products and techniques to prevent premature aging.
- Step-by-step makeup tutorials for natural and stunning looks.
- Strength exercises that boost metabolism and shape the body.
- Yoga and flexibility exercises that improve posture and mental clarity.
- Nutritional tips to nourish your body and enhance your physical appearance.

We'll also debunk common myths about beauty and fitness, so you can make informed decisions that truly fit your body and lifestyle. By the end of this journey, you'll be equipped with the knowledge to create a sustainable beauty and fitness routine that fits your needs and goals.

HOW TO USE THIS BOOK

Whether you're new to the world of beauty and fitness or looking to upgrade your current routine, this book is designed to meet your needs wherever you are. You can read it from start to finish or skip to the sections that interest you most. Each chapter is designed to provide comprehensive information, with key points and actionable steps you can implement right away.

Consistency is key when it comes to beauty and fitness, and this book focuses on long-term habits rather than quick fixes. Small, everyday changes can lead to big improvements over time. As you progress through this book, you'll learn that beauty and fitness aren't about perfection—they're about feeling good about yourself and living a healthy, balanced life.

CHAPTER 1: SKINCARE ROUTINE
FOR GLOWING SKIN

Healthy, radiant skin is a cornerstone of beauty, and achieving that glow is often the result of consistent, caring skincare. A well-organized skincare routine helps protect skin from environmental damage, slows down the signs of aging, and keeps skin looking smooth and youthful. In this chapter, we'll cover the essential steps to developing a morning and nighttime skincare routine, exploring the key ingredients to include based on different skin types and concerns.

THE IMPORTANCE OF SKIN CARE ROUTINE

The skin is the largest organ in the body, acting as a protective barrier against pollution, toxins, and UV rays. It is also one of the first areas to show signs of aging, stress, and fatigue. Following a good skincare routine not only keeps your skin clean and hydrated, it also helps prevent common issues like acne, dryness, fine lines, and hyperpigmentation.

There are two basic skincare routines you should follow: one for the morning and one for the evening. Each routine has its own unique purpose: the morning routine prepares your skin for the day, while the night routine focuses on repairing and renewing your skin while you sleep.

MORNING SKIN CARE ROUTINE

T he main goal of your morning skincare routine is to protect your skin from environmental damage, such as pollution and UV rays. This routine focuses on hydration, protection, and preparation for the next day. Here are the basic steps you should follow.

1. Cleaner

- **Purpose** : Morning cleansing helps remove any oil, dirt, or bacteria that may have built up overnight.
- **How to choose** : Choose a gentle, sulfate-free cleanser that won't strip your skin of its natural oils. For dry or sensitive skin, look for hydrating cleansers with ingredients like glycerin or ceramides. For oily or acne-prone skin, a gel cleanser with salicylic acid can help control excess oil.
- **How to use** : Use lukewarm water with a small amount of cleanser. Gently massage your skin for 30 seconds before rinsing.

2. Ink

- **Purpose** : Toner helps balance the skin's pH, remove any remaining traces of dirt or oil, and prepare the skin for better absorption of other products.
- **How to choose** : An alcohol-free toner with hydrating ingredients like rose water, aloe vera, or hyaluronic acid is the best choice. For oily or acne-prone skin, choose a toner with exfoliating ingredients like salicylic acid or witch hazel.
- **How to use** : Apply the toner using a cotton pad or simply spread it on your skin with your hands.

3. Serum

- **Purpose** : Serums contain concentrated active ingredients designed to target specific skin concerns, such as dullness, hyperpigmentation, fine lines, or acne.
- **How to choose** : In the morning, a vitamin C serum is great for its antioxidant properties, which protect against free radicals and improve skin radiance. For dry skin, consider a serum with hyaluronic acid to boost hydration.
- **How to use** : Apply 2-3 drops to your face and gently press into the skin.

4. Moisturizer

- **Purpose** : Moisturizers hydrate and lock in moisture to keep skin plump and soft all day long.
- **How to choose** : For oily skin, choose a light, oil-free moisturizer. For dry skin, choose a cream rich in ingredients such as ceramides or shea butter.
- **How to use** : Apply a dime-sized amount and gently massage into your skin, focusing on dry areas.

5. Sunscreen

- **Purpose** : Using sunscreen is the most important step in any morning routine. It protects your skin from harmful UV rays, which can cause premature aging, hyperpigmentation, and even skin cancer.

- **How to choose** : Choose a broad-spectrum sunscreen with an SPF of 30 or higher. Mineral sunscreens that contain zinc oxide or titanium dioxide are ideal for sensitive skin.
- **How to use** : Apply a generous amount to all exposed skin areas, including face, neck and hands. Reapply every two hours if spending time outdoors.

NIGHT SKIN CARE ROUTINE

Your nighttime skincare routine focuses on repairing your skin and providing intense hydration. At night, your skin goes into rejuvenation mode, making it the perfect time to address skin concerns like aging, acne, and hyperpigmentation.

1. Cleaner

- **Purpose** : Nightly cleansing is essential to remove makeup, dirt, oil and pollutants that have accumulated throughout the day.
- **How to choose** : Double cleansing at night is highly recommended, especially if you wear makeup. Start with an oil-based cleanser to break down makeup and sunscreen, then follow with a gentle water-based cleanser.
- **How to use** : Massage the oil cleanser onto dry skin, then rinse with water. Use a water-based cleanser to remove any residue.

2. Scrub (2-3 times a week)

- **Purpose** : Exfoliation helps remove dead skin cells, which enhances the smoothness and radiance of the skin. It can also prevent clogged pores and acne.
- **How to choose** : Chemical exfoliants such as alpha hydroxy acids (glycolic acid, lactic acid) or beta hydroxy acids (salicylic acid) are gentler and more effective than physical exfoliants. Use a chemical exfoliant according to your skin type.
- **How to use** : After cleansing, apply chemical exfoliant with a cotton pad or as directed. Avoid using it every night to avoid irritation.

3. Serum

- **Purpose** : At night, you can use more targeted treatments. For anti-aging, retinol or peptides can stimulate collagen production and reduce wrinkles. For hyperpigmentation, consider niacinamide or alpha arbutin.
- **How to choose** : Use a serum that suits your specific skin concern. Retinol is ideal for aging skin, while niacinamide works well for red, acne-prone skin.
- **How to use** : Apply a few drops and gently press onto your skin after exfoliating or cleansing.

4. Moisturizer

- **Purpose** : At night, a heavy moisturizer helps repair the skin barrier and lock in moisture.
- **How to choose** : Choose a rich night cream or hydrating mask that contains ingredients like ceramides, squalane, or hyaluronic acid to hydrate your skin throughout the night.
- **How to use** : Apply a generous amount and massage it on your face and neck.

5. Eye cream

- **Purpose** : The skin around your eyes is thin and prone to fine lines and dark circles. An eye cream can hydrate the area and reduce puffiness or wrinkles.
- **How to choose** : Look for eye creams that contain ingredients like caffeine (for dark circles and puffiness) or peptides (for firming and anti-aging).
- **How to use** : Gently spread a small amount under your eyes using your ring finger.

MAIN INGREDIENTS IN SKIN CARE PRODUCTS

Understanding the key ingredients in your skincare products is essential to tailoring your skincare routine to your needs. Here are some of the most effective ingredients to look for:

- **Hyaluronic Acid** : A hydrating powerhouse that attracts moisture to the skin, making it ideal for all skin types, especially dry or dehydrated skin.
- **Vitamin C** : A powerful antioxidant that works to lighten the skin, fade dark spots, and protect against environmental damage.
- **Retinol** : A derivative of Vitamin A, retinol is known for its anti-aging benefits, improving skin texture, and reducing fine lines and wrinkles.
- **Niacinamide** : This versatile ingredient helps treat redness, acne, and pigmentation while also improving skin texture.
- **Alpha Hydroxy Acids (AHAs) and Beta Hydroxy Acids (BHAs)** : Exfoliating acids that help remove dead skin cells, unclog pores, and reveal smoother, brighter skin.
- **Ceramides** : Essential for maintaining the skin's moisture barrier, and great for dry and sensitive skin types.
- **Sunscreen** : Look for mineral sunscreens that contain zinc oxide or titanium dioxide for broad-spectrum protection against both UVA and UVB rays.

CHAPTER TWO: ANTI-AGING TIPS AND PRODUCTS

Aging is a natural part of life, and while we can't stop the clock, we can certainly slow down its visible effects. Fine lines, wrinkles, sagging skin, and age spots are often the first signs of aging skin. Fortunately, with the right anti-aging routine, it's possible to maintain youthful, radiant skin for longer. In this chapter, we'll explore some of the most effective anti-aging tips and products, focusing on prevention and treatment.

UNDERSTANDING SKIN AGING

As we age, our skin undergoes many changes:

- **Loss of collagen and elastin** : Collagen and elastin are proteins that give skin its firmness and elasticity. After the age of 25, production of these proteins declines, leading to the appearance of fine lines and wrinkles.
- **Thinning skin** : Over time, the outer layer of skin (epidermis) becomes thinner, making the skin more susceptible to damage and decreased moisture retention.
- **Slow cell renewal** : As we age, the skin's ability to shed dead skin cells and regenerate new ones decreases, leading to dullness and uneven texture.
- **Environmental Damage** : Exposure to UV rays, pollution and free radicals accelerates the aging process, causing premature aging, pigmentation and rough texture.

The goal of anti-aging skin care is to minimize these changes and protect your skin from further damage. Consistency is key, and the earlier you start incorporating anti-aging habits, the more effective they will be.

1. SUN PROTECTION: THE ULTIMATE ANTI-AGING PRACTICE

Sun protection is one of the most important components of any anti-aging routine. Ultraviolet rays are one of the main causes of premature aging, known as photoaging . UVA rays penetrate deeply into the skin and break down collagen and elastin, leading to wrinkles and sagging skin.

Sunscreen

- **Why it's important** : Using sunscreen daily is the most effective way to prevent wrinkles, sun spots, and skin cancer.
- **Best Practices** : Choose a broad-spectrum sunscreen with an SPF of at least 30 that protects against both UVA and UVB rays. Apply generously to all exposed areas, including your face, neck, and hands, and reapply every two hours if you're outdoors.
- **Best Products** :
  - **EltaMD UV Clear Broad-Spectrum SPF 46** : A lightweight, oil-free sunscreen that works well for sensitive and acne-prone skin. Contains niacinamide to calm redness.
  - **Neutrogena Ultra Sheer Dry Touch SPF 70** : Provides high sun protection with a matte finish, suitable for oily skin types.

2. RETINOL: THE GOLD STANDARD FOR ANTI-AGING

Retinol, a derivative of vitamin A, is one of the most effective ingredients in anti-aging skincare. It works to promote cell turnover and stimulate collagen production, helping to reduce the appearance of fine lines, wrinkles, and dark spots.

Why does retinol work?

- **Promotes cell renewal** : Retinol accelerates the shedding of dead skin cells and the production of new cells, resulting in smoother, younger-looking skin.
- **Collagen production** : By stimulating collagen, retinol helps hydrate the skin, reducing the depth of wrinkles.
- **Improve skin texture** : Regular use of retinol can help reduce the appearance of pores, even out skin tone, and improve overall texture.

How to use retinol

- **Start Slow** : If you're new to using retinol, start by using it two to three times a week to avoid skin irritation. You can increase the frequency of use as your skin builds up tolerance.
- **Nighttime use** : Retinol makes your skin more sensitive to the sun, so it's best to use it at night. Always follow up with sunscreen during the day.
- **Moisturize the skin** : Retinol can be drying, so it is essential to use a rich moisturizer to keep the skin hydrated.

Best Products:

- **The Ordinary Retinol 0.5% in Squalane** : A budget-friendly option that combines retinol and squalane to combat dryness.
- **SkinCeuticals Retinol 0.5 Purifying Night Cream** : A powerful retinol cream with added botanical extracts to soothe skin and reduce irritation.

3. ANTIOXIDANTS: FIGHT FREE RADICALS

Free radicals are unstable molecules that can damage skin cells, leading to premature aging. They are primarily caused by environmental factors such as UV rays, pollution, and smoking. Antioxidants neutralize free radicals and help protect the skin from oxidative stress.

Vitamin C

- **Benefits** : Vitamin C is a powerful antioxidant that works to lighten the skin, reduce pigmentation, and boost collagen production. It also protects the skin from free radical damage caused by UV rays.
- **How to use** : Apply Vitamin C Serum in the morning before moisturizer and sunscreen for extra protection.
- **Best Products** :
  - **SkinCeuticals CE Ferulic** : A highly effective antioxidant serum with a blend of Vitamin C, E and Ferulic Acid for maximum protection and radiance.
  - **La Roche-Posay Pure Vitamin C Serum for Face** : A more cost-effective option that helps reduce the appearance of fine lines and even out skin tone.

Vitamin E

- **Benefits** : Vitamin E is an antioxidant that helps repair skin damage and moisturize dry skin. It works well with Vitamin C, as each enhances the effectiveness of the other.
- **How to use** : Look for products that combine vitamins C and E, as they provide stronger protection when used together.

Green tea extract

- **Benefits** : Green tea extract is rich in polyphenols, which help reduce inflammation and neutralize free radicals.
- **How to Use** : Skincare products containing green tea, such as serums or creams, are ideal for soothing sensitive or irritated skin while providing antioxidant benefits.
- **Best Product : Paula's Choice Super Antioxidant Concentrate** : Contains green tea extract, vitamin C, and peptides for comprehensive anti-aging care.

4. MOISTURIZING: THE KEY TO PLUMP, YOUTHFUL SKIN

As we age, our skin loses its ability to retain moisture, leading to dryness, fine lines, and dull skin. Proper hydration is essential to keeping skin plump and firm, which is why hydration should be an essential part of any anti-aging routine.

hyaluronic acid

- **Benefits** : Hyaluronic acid is a humectant, meaning it attracts moisture to the skin and holds it there. It can hold up to 1,000 times its weight in water, making it an excellent moisturizing ingredient for all skin types.
- **How to use** : Apply hyaluronic acid serum or moisturizer after cleansing to lock in hydration.
- **Best Products** :
  - **The Ordinary Hyaluronic Acid 2% + B5** : A budget-friendly option that provides intense hydration with added vitamin B5 to soothe skin.
  - **Neutrogena Hydro Boost Water Gel** : A lightweight gel moisturizer with hyaluronic acid, ideal for daily hydration.

Ceramides

- **Benefits** : Ceramides are fatty acids that help restore the skin's natural barrier and prevent moisture loss. As we age, our skin produces less ceramides, so replenishing them is essential to keep skin hydrated and youthful.
- **How to use** : Look for moisturizers and night creams that contain ceramides, especially if you have dry or sensitive skin.
- **Best Product : CeraVe Moisturizing Cream** : Rich in ceramides and hyaluronic acid, this cream is ideal for restoring the skin barrier and locking in moisture.

5. ANTI-AGING LIFESTYLE HABITS

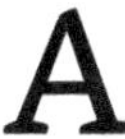

long with skin care products, lifestyle factors play a significant role in how our skin ages. Making healthy choices can slow down the aging process and improve the overall appearance of your skin.

Sleep

- **Benefits** : While you sleep, your skin goes into repair mode, producing new collagen and repairing damage. Make sure you get 7-9 hours of good sleep each night to wake up with refreshed skin.
- **Tip** : Sleeping on your back and using a silk pillowcase can reduce friction and prevent sleep lines.

Diet

- **Benefits** : A diet rich in antioxidants, vitamins, and omega-3 fatty acids can support skin health from the inside out. Foods like berries, leafy greens, nuts, and fatty fish provide the nutrients your skin needs to stay healthy and youthful.
- **Tip** : Keep your body hydrated by drinking plenty of water throughout the day, and reduce your intake of sugar and processed foods, which can speed up the aging process.

Practice

- **Benefits** : Regular exercise improves circulation, delivering more oxygen and nutrients to the skin. It also helps reduce stress, which is known to contribute to aging.
- **Tip** : Incorporate cardio and strength training into your routine for optimal skin and overall health benefits.

CHAPTER 3: MAKEUP TIPS FOR A NATURAL LOOK

The "natural look" has become one of the hottest beauty trends in recent years. It focuses on enhancing your features rather than hiding them, creating the illusion of fresh, glowing skin without looking overdone. The key to this approach is using the right techniques and products to achieve a flawless finish that looks effortless. In this chapter, we'll walk you through the steps needed to create a natural makeup look, focusing on subtle enhancements to your skin, eyes, and lips.

1. SKIN PREPARATION: THE FOUNDATION OF A NATURAL LOOK

Before applying makeup, it is essential to make sure that your skin is well prepared. Soft, moisturized skin will not only make your makeup last longer, but will also ensure that it looks natural and radiant.

Skin care before makeup

- **Moisturize** : Start by moisturizing your skin to ensure it is plump and smooth. Choose a lightweight, hydrating moisturizer that absorbs quickly and leaves no residue.
- **Primer** : Primer helps create an even surface for makeup application while ensuring that foundation stays in place. Choose a hydrating or matte primer based on your skin type.
  - **Tip** : If you have large pores, use a primer to fill in pores in specific areas such as the T-zone.

Best Products:

- **Embryolisse Lait-Crème Concentré** : A favorite moisturizer that gives skin a smooth base for makeup.
- **Smashbox Photo Finish Primer** : A lightweight primer that helps hide imperfections and extend the wear of foundation.

2. GET FLAWLESS SKIN USING MINIMAL PRODUCTS.

The natural look starts with a focus on the skin, creating an even, radiant complexion without overusing products. The goal is to let your natural skin shine through while subtly correcting imperfections.

Foundation or tinted moisturizer?

- **Tinted Moisturizer/BB Cream** : For a super natural look, opt for a tinted moisturizer or BB cream. These products provide light coverage while adding hydration and a dewy finish to the skin. They're perfect for evening out your skin tone without looking heavy.
- **Foundation** : If you prefer more coverage, choose a lightweight, buildable foundation. Look for formulas that mimic your natural skin texture, such as sheer or light coverage foundations with a luminous finish.
    - **Tip** : Apply foundation sparingly—only where you need it (e.g., around your nose, chin, and any red areas). Use a damp beauty sponge or foundation brush to blend it in for an airbrushed effect.

Concealer for specific coverage

- **Purpose** : Use concealer to brighten the under-eye area, cover blemishes, or hide discoloration. Choose a lightweight concealer that won't crease or look too thick.
- **How to use** : Apply a small amount of concealer under your eyes in a triangle shape and over any blemishes or dark spots. Blend using your fingers or a small brush for a seamless finish.
    - **Tip** : When it comes to concealing imperfections, less is better than more. Avoid applying too much product, which can result in a cakey look.

Best Products:

- **NARS Pure Radiant Tinted Moisturizer** : Provides light coverage with a natural, radiant finish.
- **IT Cosmetics Your Skin But Better CC+ Cream** : A full-coverage BB cream that hydrates and corrects imperfections.
- **Maybelline Fit Me Concealer** : A lightweight, affordable option that provides great coverage without looking heavy.

3. BLUSH AND BRONZER: ADD SUBTLE DIMENSIONS

For a natural look, blush and bronzer are essential to give your skin a warm, healthy glow. The idea is to enhance your skin's natural flush and create a sun-kissed look without harsh lines or over-the-top color.

blush

- **Cream vs. Powder Blush** : Cream blush is great for a natural, dewy look because it melts into the skin and mimics the texture of natural skin. Powder blush is better for oily skin or if you prefer a matte finish.
- **How to use** : Smile and gently apply blush to the apples of your cheeks, blending out toward your temples. Use your fingers or a sponge for cream blush and a fluffy brush for powder.
    - o **Tip** : Stick to soft, natural colors like peach, coral, or soft pink for a natural-looking red.

Bronzer

- **Purpose** : Bronzer adds warmth and dimension to your face, giving you a sun-kissed glow. Choose a matte bronzer for a natural look or a bronzer with a subtle shimmer for a luminous finish.
- **How to use** : Gently apply bronzer to areas of your face that are naturally exposed to the sun - your forehead, cheekbones and jawline. Use a large, fluffy brush and blend well for a seamless look.
    - o **Tip** : Avoid using a bronzer that is too dark; the goal is to achieve a naturally warm look, not an overly tanned one.

Best Products:

- **Glossier Cloud Paint (Blush)** : A creamy gel blush that gives you a natural, sheer glow.
- **Milk Makeup Matte Bronzer** : A creamy bronzer that blends seamlessly for a natural look.
- **Benefit Hoola Bronzer** : A classic matte bronzer that works well for a soft, sun-kissed look.

4. EYE MAKEUP: PRECISE DEFINITION

For a natural look, your eye makeup should enhance your eyes without overdoing it. Stick to neutral colors, soft lines, and simple layers for a fresh, conscious look.

Eyebrows

- **Purpose** : Well-groomed brows instantly define the face and enhance your natural look. For soft, natural-looking brows, focus on filling in sparse areas without creating overly defined lines.
- **How to use** : Use an eyebrow pencil or powder that matches your natural brow color. Gently fill in any gaps using short, hair-like strokes. Brush with a small brush to soften edges and blend product.
    - o **Tip** : Avoid harsh, clumpy brows to achieve this look. Keep them soft and natural.

eye shadow

- **Neutral Colors** : Stick to neutral, earthy tones like beige, tan, or soft brown. The goal is to add subtle depth and brightness without using dramatic colors.
- **How to use** : Apply a light neutral shade to your eyelids and use a slightly darker shade to define the crease of the eyelid. Blend well for a smooth, natural color gradient.
    - o **Tip** : You can skip the eyeshadow altogether and apply a little bronzer to your eyelids for a cohesive, natural look.

Mascara

- **Length and definition** : Mascara helps open up your eyes and make them look more awake. Choose a lengthening or defining mascara that separates your lashes and avoids clumps.
- **How to use** : Curl your lashes first to lift and highlight your eyes. Then apply a light coat of mascara to the upper and lower lashes, swishing the wand at the base for maximum definition.
    - o **Tip** : For a more natural look, choose brown mascara instead of black.

Best Products:

- **Anastasia Beverly Hills Brow Wiz** : A precise eyebrow pencil perfect for creating natural, hair-like strokes.
- **Urban Decay Naked Basics Eyeshadow Palette** : A collection of neutral shades perfect for everyday use.
- **L'Oreal Lash Paradise Mascara** : A volumizing mascara that defines and lengthens lashes without clumping.

5. LIPS: SOFT AND NATURAL

For a natural makeup look, lips should appear soft, moisturized and subtly enhanced. The goal is to highlight your natural lip color rather than create a bold look.

Lip balm or tinted lip balm

- **Moisturize first** : Start by applying lip balm to keep your lips soft and smooth.
- **Tinted Lip Balm** : For a little color, use a tinted lip balm that adds a natural flush to your lips while keeping them moisturized.
  - **Tip** : Choose a color close to your natural lip color, such as soft pink, peach, or beige.

lipstick or lip gloss

- **Sheer formulas** : If you prefer more color, use a sheer lipstick or lip gloss. Sheer formulas give you a hint of color without the heaviness of a full-coverage lipstick.
- **How to use** : Gently apply lipstick to your lips and blend with your fingers for a smooth, natural finish. The clear lip gloss adds shine without looking overdone.
  - **Tip** : Avoid matte lipstick for this look, as it may make your lips look heavy or dry.

Best Products:

- **Fresh Sugar Tinted Lip Treatment** : A moisturizing tinted balm that comes in a variety of natural-looking shades.
- **Glossier Generation G Sheer Matte Lipstick** : A sheer lipstick that gives your lips a natural finish.
- **Burt's Bees Tinted Lip Balm** : An affordable, moisturizing lip balm with a hint of color.

FINISHING TOUCHES: SETTING MAKEUP

To ensure your natural makeup stays put all day, finish with a setting spray or a light dusting of translucent powder. If you prefer a dewy finish, a hydrating mist will lock in moisture and keep your skin looking fresh. For oily skin, a translucent powder will help control shine without adding any extra color.

Best Products:

- **Urban Decay All Nighter Setting Spray** : Keeps makeup in place all day without feeling heavy or dry.
- **Laura Mercier Translucent Setting Powder** : A cult favorite that sets makeup with a natural, matte finish.

CHAPTER FOUR: HAIR CARE AND HAIRSTYLES

Hair is often considered the "glory of a person," and just like skin, healthy hair requires regular care and attention. A good hair care routine helps maintain the natural vibrancy of your hair, whether it is long or short, curly or straight. This chapter will cover basic tips for maintaining healthy hair and some easy hairstyles that you can incorporate into your daily routine.

1. UNDERSTAND YOUR HAIR TYPE

Before creating a hair care routine, it's important to understand your hair type. Your hair type affects which products and techniques will work best for you. Here are some common hair types:

- **Straight hair** : It is often smooth and shiny but can get greasy quickly.
- **Wavy hair** : Has a slight curl or wave, and may be prone to frizz.
- **Curly hair** : has defined curls or waves that can be prone to dryness and frizz.
- **Curly/wavy hair** : has tight curls or coils and is often drier due to its natural texture.

Once you know your hair type, you can tailor your routine to meet specific needs, like hydration for dry curls or volume for fine, straight hair.

2. DAILY HAIR CARE ROUTINE

Following a regular hair care routine is essential to keeping your hair healthy and strong. Here is a basic daily routine that can be modified to suit any hair type.

disinfection

- **Frequency** : How often you wash your hair depends on your hair type. If you have oily hair, you may need to wash it every day or every other day. For dry or curly hair, washing it two to three times a week is usually enough to avoid stripping the hair of its natural oils.
- **Shampoo** : Choose a sulfate-free shampoo that cleanses your hair without drying it out. Sulfates can strip your scalp of natural oils, leading to dryness, especially for curly or wavy hair.
  - o **Tip** : Focus on the scalp when shampooing, as this is where oils and dirt accumulate. Let the shampoo run through your hair strands to clean the rest of your hair without over-washing it.

conditioning

- **Purpose** : Conditioner helps moisturize and detangle hair, making it easier to style. It also smooths the hair cuticle, reducing frizz and adding shine.
- **How to use** : Apply conditioner to mid-lengths and ends of your hair, avoiding the roots to prevent greasiness. Leave on for 2-5 minutes before rinsing.
  - o **Tip** : If your hair is very dry or damaged, use a leave-in conditioner or deep conditioning treatment once a week for extra hydration.

Best Products:

- **Sulfate free shampoo** :
  - o **SheaMoisture Coconut & Hibiscus Curl & Shine Shampoo** : Ideal for curly and dry hair types, it moisturizes without stripping away natural oils.
  - o **L'Oreal Paris EverPure Moisture Shampoo** : A sulfate-free, budget-friendly shampoo that's safe for color-treated hair.
- **Balm** :
  - o **Australian Miracle 3 Minute Deep Conditioner** : Deep conditioner that works in just three minutes.
  - o **Moroccanoil Hydrating Conditioner** : Adds moisture and shine, especially to dry or chemically treated hair.

3. HAIR CARE AND STYLING

After washing and styling your hair, how you treat and style your hair can affect its long-term health. Overuse of heat or failure to protect your hair from environmental damage can cause breakage, dryness, and dullness. Here are some tips for caring for and styling your hair after washing.

detangle

- **How to detangle** : Wet hair is more prone to breakage, so it's important to handle it gently. Use a wide-toothed comb or detangling brush to remove tangles from the ends to the roots. Avoid using regular brushes on wet hair, as they can pull it and cause breakage.
  - **Tip** : Apply a leave-in conditioner or detangling spray to help loosen knots and make the detangling process smoother.

Heat styling

- **Heat Protection** : If you use heat tools like a blow dryer, flat iron, or curling iron, always apply a heat protectant spray to your hair beforehand. This creates a barrier that helps reduce heat damage.
- **How to minimize heat damage** : To avoid overexposure to heat, let your hair air dry whenever possible or use the "cool" setting on your blow dryer. If you must use heat tools, try to limit them to once or twice a week.
  - **Tip** : Consider investing in ceramic or tourmaline heat tools, which distribute heat more evenly and are gentle on hair.

Best Products:

- **Heat protector** :
  - **TRESemmé Thermal Creations Heat Tamer Spray** : A lightweight, affordable option that protects hair from heat damage.
  - **Living Proof Restore Instant Protection** : Heat and UV protector provides extra shine and protects hair from environmental stressors.

4. EASY HAIRSTYLES FOR EVERY DAY

Sometimes, all you need is a simple hairstyle to enhance your look and add some stylish touches to your overall look. Here are some easy hairstyles that suit most hair types.

low bun

- **How to do it** : The low bun is a classic, elegant hairstyle that's perfect for both casual and formal occasions. Start by gathering your hair at the nape of your neck, then twist it into a bun and secure it with a hair tie or bobby pins. Pull out a few strands that frame your face to soften the look.
  - **Tip** : For a polished finish, smooth any flyaway hairs with a light-hold hairspray.

loose waves

- **How to make it** : Loose waves give you a relaxed, beachy look. If your hair is naturally wavy or curly, you can enhance its natural texture by applying a curl enhancing cream and curling your hair while it is damp. For straight hair, use a curling iron or flat iron to create soft waves by wrapping sections of hair around the barrel.
  - **Tip** : After curling your hair, gently run your fingers through the waves to break them up and create a more natural, tousled effect.

top knot

- **How to do it** : A top knot is an easy and simple hairstyle that's great for days when you're short on time. Gather your hair into a high ponytail at the crown of your head, then twist the ponytail and wrap your hair into a bun. Secure with a hair tie or bobby pins.
  - **Tip** : For extra volume, backcomb the hair at the crown of your head before gathering it into a ponytail.

elegant ponytail

- **How to do it** : A sleek ponytail is a versatile hairstyle that works for day or night. Comb your hair back and secure it in a high or low ponytail with a hair tie. Use a small amount of gel or serum to smooth out any frizz or flyaways for a sleek finish.
  - **Tip** : For a more polished look, take a small section of hair from the ponytail and wrap it around the hair tie to hide it.

Best hair styling products:

- **Curl enhancing cream** :
  - **Ouai Curl Crème** : A lightweight cream that defines curls while adding moisture and shine.
- **Hairspray** :
  - **L'Oreal Paris Elnett Satin Hairspray** : A flexible hairspray that controls frizz without making your hair stiff.

5. PROTECT YOUR HAIR: LONG-TERM CARE

Healthy hair is the result of consistent care, which includes protecting it from damage. Here are some long-term tips to keep your hair looking its best.

Trim regularly

- **Why it's important** : Regular trims are essential to prevent split ends and keep your hair healthy. Even if you grow your hair out, trimming it every 8 to 12 weeks will help maintain its shape and prevent breakage.

Protection from sun damage

- **UV Protection** : Just like your skin, your hair can be damaged by the sun's UV rays. Prolonged exposure to the sun can dry out, discolor, and weaken your hair. Use a UV protection spray or wear a hat when spending time outdoors.
  - **Tip** : Look for hair products that contain UV filters to protect your hair from environmental damage.

Reduce chemical treatments

- **Why it's important** : Frequent chemical treatments like dyeing, perming, or straightening can weaken your hair and lead to breakage. If you color or treat your hair regularly, be sure to follow up with deep conditioning treatments to restore moisture and strength.

Best product:

- **UV protection** :
  - **Aveda Sunscreen Hair Protectant** : A lightweight, water-resistant spray that provides UV protection.

CHAPTER FIVE: COMPREHENSIVE BEAUTY

True beauty is not just about skincare and makeup, it's about nourishing the mind, body, and spirit. Holistic beauty emphasizes that everything from the food you eat to how you manage stress and sleep affects your outward appearance. In this chapter, we'll explore the role of hydration, sleep, and self-care in maintaining a radiant, youthful appearance.

1. MOISTURIZING: THE FOUNDATION OF GLOWING SKIN

Hydration is one of the simplest and most effective ways to achieve naturally glowing skin. Our bodies are made up of about 60% water, and staying hydrated helps maintain skin elasticity, improve circulation, and remove toxins. On the other hand, dehydration can cause skin to appear dry, dull, and more prone to wrinkles.

Why is hydration important for beauty?

- **Maintains Skin Elasticity** : Well-hydrated skin looks fuller and younger because it maintains its elasticity. Dry skin is more prone to fine lines and rough texture.
- **Detoxification** : Drinking enough water helps flush toxins from your system, which may reduce the likelihood of skin problems like acne and inflammation.
- **Improves skin** : Proper hydration helps improve blood circulation, giving your skin a healthy glow and reducing puffiness or bags under the eyes.

How much water should you drink?

The general recommendation is to drink about 8 cups (64 ounces) of water per day, but this may vary depending on factors such as activity level, climate, and individual needs. To make sure you stay hydrated:

- **Listen to your body** : Drink when you feel thirsty, and try to have water with every meal.
- **Add hydrating foods** : Include water-rich foods in your diet, such as cucumbers, watermelons, oranges, and leafy greens, which help boost hydration levels.

Tip: If you have trouble drinking enough water, try flavoring it with slices of fruit, herbs like mint, or a squeeze of lemon for a more refreshing and enjoyable drink.

2. THE RELATIONSHIP BETWEEN SLEEP AND BEAUTY

"Beauty sleep" isn't just a saying. When you sleep, your body goes into repair mode, renewing skin cells and producing collagen, a protein that's essential for keeping skin firm and preventing wrinkles. Getting enough sleep is crucial to looking and feeling your best, as lack of sleep can lead to dull skin, dark circles, and increased stress hormones, which can worsen skin conditions like acne or eczema.

How Sleep Affects Your Skin

- **Collagen Production** : During deep sleep, the body increases collagen production, which helps keep skin firm and elastic. Lack of sleep can lead to decreased collagen levels, leading to sagging skin and more visible wrinkles.
- **Cell Renewal** : While you sleep, your skin cells regenerate, allowing damaged cells to be repaired. This process helps maintain clear, even-toned skin.
- **Dark circles and puffiness** : Lack of sleep can lead to fluid retention, which causes puffiness, especially around the eyes. It can also increase the appearance of dark circles.

Tips for better sleep and better beauty

- **Create a nighttime routine** : Try going to bed at the same time each night and creating a calming routine before bed, such as reading or meditation, to signal to your body that it's time to wind down.
- **Invest in silk pillowcases** : Silk pillowcases are gentler on skin and hair than cotton, reducing friction that can lead to sleep lines and hair breakage.
- **Sleeping on your back** : Sleeping on your back helps prevent pressure on the face, which may reduce the development of wrinkles.

3. SELF-CARE RITUALS FOR INNER AND OUTER BEAUTY

Self-care is essential to maintaining emotional and physical health, and it directly impacts how we look and feel. When we take the time to care for ourselves, it reduces stress, improves our mood, and contributes to a more radiant and glowing appearance. Incorporating simple self-care rituals into your daily routine can help promote balance and beauty from within.

Mindfulness and meditation

- **Stress and its effects on the skin** : Stress releases the hormone cortisol, which can lead to inflammation, breakouts, and premature aging. Practicing mindfulness and meditation can help reduce stress levels, promote clearer skin, and a more peaceful state of mind.
- **Meditation for Beauty** : Studies have shown that meditation can reduce stress hormones and improve sleep quality, both of which have a direct impact on your skin. Even just 10 minutes of mindful meditation a day can help you manage stress and feel more balanced.

Aromatherapy

- **Benefits for Skin and Mood** : Aromatherapy can be a powerful tool in promoting relaxation and improving overall health. Essential oils such as lavender, chamomile, and rose have calming properties that can soothe the skin and mind.
- **How to use** : Add a few drops of essential oils to an aromatherapy diffuser, or apply diluted oils to your wrists or temples for a calming effect throughout the day.

Spa days at home

- **Pamper your skin** : Every now and then, make time for a spa day at home. Use a face mask, take a long bath, and apply a nourishing body oil to relax and rejuvenate your skin.
- **Tip** : Try using a homemade mask made with natural ingredients like honey, yogurt, or avocado for a moisturizing and soothing treatment.

4. EAT FOR BEAUTY: NOURISHMENT FROM THE INSIDE OUT

What you put in your body is just as important as what you put on your skin when it comes to beauty. A nutrient-rich diet can have a huge impact on the health and appearance of your skin, hair, and nails. Certain foods contain vitamins and minerals that help promote healthy skin, strong hair, and healthy nails.

Essential nutrients that enhance beauty

- **Vitamin C** : Essential for collagen production, vitamin C helps keep skin firm and youthful. Foods rich in vitamin C include oranges, strawberries, bell peppers, and spinach.
- **Omega-3 fatty acids** : Omega-3 fatty acids are found in foods such as salmon, chia seeds, and walnuts, and help reduce inflammation and keep skin hydrated.
- **Biotin (Vitamin B7)** : Biotin is known for its ability to promote healthy hair and nails. You can find it in foods like eggs, nuts, and sweet potatoes.
- **Antioxidants** : Antioxidants help protect the skin from damage caused by free radicals, which contribute to premature aging. Foods rich in antioxidants include berries, dark chocolate, and green tea.

Tip: Include a variety of fruits and vegetables in your diet to ensure you get a variety of skin-boosting vitamins and minerals.

5. BALANCE MIND, BODY AND SPIRIT FOR RADIANT BEAUTY.

Holistic beauty isn't just about taking care of your physical appearance; it's about fostering harmony between mind, body, and spirit. When you feel good on the inside, it shows on the outside. Practices that help balance mental and emotional health are just as important to your beauty as skincare or makeup.

Yoga and movement

- **Physical Benefits** : Yoga improves flexibility, strength, and posture, all of which contribute to a fitter appearance. Regular movement also promotes blood circulation, delivering more oxygen and nutrients to the skin for a healthy glow.
- **Mental Benefits** : Yoga and other forms of exercise reduce stress, improve mood, and promote mental clarity. These benefits not only enhance your overall health, but also contribute to clearer skin and a more youthful appearance.

Positive thinking and self-love

- **The Power of Positive Thinking** : How you feel about yourself directly affects how you present yourself to the world. Cultivating a positive mindset and practicing self-love can change the way you look and feel.
- **Beauty Affirmations** : Practice daily affirmations like "I am beautiful inside and out" or "I am worthy of care and love." These simple phrases can help you embrace your unique beauty and build confidence over time.

CHAPTER 6: FITNESS BASICS

Fitness is the cornerstone of a healthy lifestyle, playing a crucial role in promoting inner health and outer beauty. Following a regular fitness routine not only helps you maintain a healthy weight, but it also improves your skin, boosts energy levels, and enhances your mental health. In this chapter, we'll explain the basics of fitness, discuss the different types of exercise, and guide you through setting realistic fitness goals.

1. WHY IS FITNESS ESSENTIAL FOR BEAUTY AND HEALTH?

Fitness is not just about aesthetics, it's about building strength, endurance, and flexibility that support overall body function. A well-rounded fitness routine can have multiple benefits for your health, including:

- **Improves Circulation** : Exercise increases blood flow, delivering more oxygen and nutrients to your skin and other vital organs. This improved circulation promotes a glowing complexion and helps detoxify your skin.
- **Better Sleep** : Regular physical activity helps regulate sleep patterns, leading to better quality rest, which is essential for skin repair and mental health.
- **Mental health benefits** : Exercise releases endorphins, the body's natural feel-good chemicals that help reduce stress, anxiety, and depression. A balanced mind also promotes clear, healthy skin and a more positive outlook on life.
- **Weight management** : Regular exercise helps maintain a healthy body weight, which may improve confidence and reduce the risk of various chronic diseases.
- **Stronger muscles and bones** : Strength training and weight-bearing exercises help maintain muscle mass and bone density, which are essential for posture, balance, and longevity.

2. THE FIVE COMPONENTS OF PHYSICAL FITNESS

To achieve overall fitness, it is important to include a variety of exercises that target different areas of the body. The five main components of fitness are:

- **Cardiorespiratory capacity** : Refers to the efficiency of the heart and lungs in delivering oxygen to the muscles during prolonged physical activity. Activities such as running, cycling, and swimming improve this capacity.
- **Muscle strength** : The amount of force a muscle can produce in a single effort. Strength exercises such as weight lifting or body weight exercises (such as push-ups and squats) help increase muscle strength.
- **Muscular endurance** : Muscular endurance is the ability of a muscle to sustain repeated contractions over time without fatigue. Exercises such as planks, lunges, and cycling build this endurance.
- **Flexibility** : Flexibility refers to the range of motion available in a joint. Stretching exercises and practices such as yoga improve flexibility, which may reduce the risk of injury and improve posture.
- **Body Composition** : Body composition is the ratio of fat to lean muscle mass in the body. Regular exercise along with a balanced diet helps maintain a healthy body composition.

Each component contributes to overall fitness and should be included in your routine for a balanced approach to health and well-being.

3. HOW TO SET REALISTIC FITNESS GOALS

One of the most common mistakes people make when starting their fitness journey is setting goals that are too ambitious or vague. To ensure long-term success, it is important to set goals that are realistic and measurable. One popular method for setting goals is the SMART method , which stands for specific, measurable, achievable, relevant, and time-bound.

Setting SMART Fitness Goals

- **Specific** : Be clear about what you want to achieve. Instead of saying, "I want to get fit," say, "I want to be able to run a 5K without stopping."
- **Measurable** : Make sure you can track your progress. For example, "I want to increase the number of push-ups I can do from 10 to 20 over the next month."
- **Achievable** : Set challenging but achievable goals. If you're new to exercise, start with smaller goals like walking for 30 minutes three times a week before progressing to more intense exercises.
- **Related** : Make sure your goals align with your personal values and what's important to you. For example, if improving your energy levels and mental health are priorities, focus on getting regular moderate exercise rather than just losing weight.
- **Time Commitment** : Set a deadline for your goals. This gives you a clear time frame to work toward and helps you stay accountable. For example, "I want to complete a 5K race in 12 weeks."

Examples of fitness goals

- **Goal for beginners** : "I want to walk briskly for 30 minutes, five days a week for the next month to improve my cardiovascular endurance."
- **Intermediate goal** : "I want to be able to do 20 push-ups in a row without stopping for the next six weeks."
- **Advanced goal** : "I want to improve my flexibility enough to do a full forward bend by the end of this year."

4. TYPES OF EXERCISES AND THEIR BENEFITS

There are different types of exercises, each with its own set of benefits. A well-rounded fitness routine should include a combination of these exercises to improve overall strength, endurance, flexibility, and balance.

Cardiovascular exercises

- **Purpose** : Cardio exercises improve heart and lung function, helping your body use oxygen more efficiently. They also burn calories and support weight loss.
- **Examples** : running, brisk walking, cycling, swimming, dancing, jumping rope.
- **Frequency** : Try to do at least 150 minutes of moderate-intensity cardio per week or 75 minutes of high-intensity cardio (eg, running, high-intensity interval training).
- **benefits** :
    - Improves heart health.
    - Boosts metabolism and helps in fat loss.
    - Enhances lung capacity and endurance.

Strength training

- **Purpose** : Strength training builds muscle, increases metabolism and improves body composition. It also helps strengthen bones and reduce the risk of injury.
- **Examples** : weight lifting, resistance band exercises, bodyweight exercises (e.g., push-ups, squats, lunges), Russian kettlebell exercises.
- **Frequency** : Try to do strength training at least two to three times a week, targeting different muscle groups in each session.
- **benefits** :
    - Increases muscle mass and strength.
    - It boosts metabolism, which helps in weight management.
    - Improves overall posture and stability.

Flexibility and mobility training

- **Purpose** : Stretching exercises increase the range of motion in joints and muscles, improving flexibility and reducing the risk of injury.
- **Examples** : yoga, Pilates, static stretching (holding a stretch for 20-30 seconds), dynamic stretching (moving through the stretch), and stretching with a foam roller.
- **Frequency** : Stretching should be done daily or at least after every exercise session. Yoga can be practiced two to three times a week.
- **benefits** :
    - Reduces muscle stiffness and pain.
    - Improve posture and flexibility.
    - Increases relaxation and reduces stress.

Balance and stability exercises

- **Purpose** : Balance training strengthens your core muscles and improves coordination, which helps prevent falls and promotes overall stability.
- **Examples** : yoga, Pilates, one-legged standing, stability ball exercises, tai chi.
- **Frequency** : Incorporate balance exercises into your routine two to three times a week.

- **benefits** :
    - Promotes coordination and core strength.
    - Improve posture and body awareness.
    - Reduces the risk of falling, especially as you age.

5. HOW TO BUILD A FITNESS ROUTINE THAT WORKS FOR YOU

Creating a fitness routine that fits your lifestyle and goals is key to sticking with it long-term. A well-rounded routine should include a balance of cardio, strength, flexibility, and balance exercises. Here's how to build a basic weekly fitness plan.

Step 1: Assess your current fitness level.

Before you begin, pay attention to your current fitness level. How often do you currently exercise? What activities do you enjoy? Are there any physical limitations that you need to take into account?

Step 2: Choose activities you enjoy.

The best fitness routine is one that you enjoy and look forward to. If you don't enjoy running, try walking, cycling, or dancing. If you don't like the gym, consider working out at home or taking group fitness classes.

Step 3: Plan your workout schedule.

Start with a realistic schedule that fits your lifestyle. Set a goal of 3-5 exercises per week, combining different types of exercises. For example:

- **Day 1** : 30 minutes of exercise (brisk walking or cycling) + 10 minutes of stretching.
- **Day 2** : Strength training (focus on upper body).
- **Day 3** : 45 minutes of yoga or Pilates.
- **Day 4** : Cardio (intermittent running or swimming) + 10 minutes of abs.
- **Day 5** : Strength training (focus on lower body).

Step 4: Track your progress

Keeping a fitness journal or using a fitness app can help you stay on track and monitor your progress. Record your workouts, how you felt, and any improvements you notice in your strength, endurance, or flexibility.

Step 5: Stay consistent.

Consistency is key to seeing results. While motivation may fluctuate, building a habit of regular exercise will keep you on track. Set small milestones and celebrate your progress along the way.

CHAPTER SEVEN: STRENGTH TRAINING FOR WOMEN

Strength training, once considered a male-dominated fitness activity, has become increasingly popular among women due to its many physical and mental benefits. Building muscle not only helps with weight management, but it also improves posture, boosts metabolism, and increases overall body confidence. In this chapter, we'll explore the benefits of strength training for women, debunk the myths surrounding weightlifting, and guide you to the best strength training exercises to build a strong, toned body.

1. BENEFITS OF STRENGTH TRAINING FOR WOMEN

Many women avoid lifting weights for fear of gaining "bulk" or excess muscle. However, strength training offers a wide range of benefits without the intense muscle growth often associated with bodybuilding. Here's why strength training should be an essential part of every woman's fitness routine.

Increase muscle strength and definition

- **Why it matters** : Strength training helps build lean muscle mass, giving your body a tight, defined look. Women have lower levels of testosterone than men, which means building big muscles is less likely, but you can still achieve a strong, sculpted look with regular strength training.
- **The result** : You will develop tight, lean arms, legs and core muscles, enhancing your overall body shape without making it bulky.

Boost metabolism

- **Why it matters** : Muscle tissue burns more calories at rest than fat tissue. This means that the more muscle you build, the more calories your body will burn throughout the day—even when you're not exercising. Strength training helps rev up your metabolism and makes it easier to maintain or lose weight.
- **The result** : You'll increase your basal metabolic rate (BMR), allowing you to burn more calories even while at rest.

improve bone density

- **Why it matters** : As women age, they become more susceptible to osteoporosis, a condition that weakens bones and increases the risk of fractures. Weight-bearing exercises such as strength training stimulate bone growth, which helps maintain bone density and reduce the risk of osteoporosis.
- **The result** : Stronger bones support long-term health and reduce the chance of injury as you age.

Improve posture and core strength

- **Why it's important** : Strengthening your muscles, especially in your core and back, improves your posture by helping you stand taller and with more confidence. Poor posture can lead to back pain and other problems, but strength training helps maintain alignment and balance in your body.
- **The result** : You will enjoy better posture, less back pain, and greater overall stability.

Mental health and confidence

- **Why it matters** : Strength training has profound effects on mental health. The sense of accomplishment that comes from lifting weights, pushing personal boundaries, and seeing physical improvements can boost your self-confidence. Strength training also releases endorphins, which are known to improve mood and reduce anxiety.
- **The result** : You will feel stronger, more capable and more confident in your body and abilities.

2. DEBUNKING MYTHS ABOUT WOMEN AND STRENGTH TRAINING

Despite the growing popularity of strength training among women, there are still many myths. Let's clear up some of the most common misconceptions.

Myth 1: Lifting weights will make you bulky.

- **Fact**: Women do not have the same hormonal makeup as men, especially lower testosterone levels, which makes it very difficult for women to build big, bulky muscles. Instead, strength training will help you build strong, lean muscles that enhance your body shape.

Myth 2: Cardiovascular exercise is better for fat loss.

- **Fact** : While cardio burns calories during your workout, strength training boosts your metabolism, helping you burn calories even after your workout is over. In fact, building muscle is one of the most effective ways to improve your body composition and lose fat.

Myth 3: Strength training is only for young women.

- **Fact** : Strength training is beneficial for women of all ages, but especially as they get older. It helps maintain muscle mass, bone density, and balance, all of which are critical to healthy aging.

Myth #4: You have to spend hours in the gym.

- **Fact** : You don't need to spend hours lifting weights to see results. Short, focused workouts with proper form and technique can be very effective. A 30-minute strength training session, done two to three times a week, can significantly improve muscle strength and overall power.

3. BEST STRENGTH EXERCISES FOR WOMEN

Strength training can be done using a variety of equipment, including dumbbells, barbells, resistance bands, and your own body weight. Here are some of the most effective exercises to build strength and tone your body.

1. Squat

- **Targeted muscles** : Quadriceps, hamstrings, glutes, core.
- **How to do it** :
  - Stand with your feet shoulder-width apart.
  - Lower your body by bending your knees and pushing your hips back as if you were sitting in a chair.
  - Keep your chest up and your knees in line with your toes.
  - Return to the starting position by pushing through your heels.
  - **Tip** : You can perform squats using just your body weight or add resistance by holding dumbbells or a barbell.

2. Stabs

- **Targeted muscles** : glutes, quadriceps, hamstrings, calves, trunk.
- **How to do it** :
  - Stand straight with your feet together.
  - Take one step forward with one foot and then lower your body until your knees are bent at a 90-degree angle.
  - Push off with your front foot to return to the starting position.
  - Repeat on the other leg.
  - **Tip** : For added resistance, hold a dumbbell in each hand while performing lunges.

3. Push-ups

- **Targeted muscles** : chest, shoulders, triceps, core.
- **How to do it** :
  - Start in a high plank position with your hands slightly wider than shoulder-width apart.
  - Lower your body toward the floor, keeping your elbows close to your body.
  - Push yourself back up to the starting position.
  - **Tip** : If regular push-ups are too difficult, you can modify them by doing push-ups on your knees or against a wall.

4. Weightlifting

- **Targeted Muscles** : Hamstrings, Glutes, Lower Back, Core.
- **How to do it** :
  - Stand with your feet hip-width apart, holding a barbell or dumbbell in front of your thighs.
  - Bend at your hips, keeping a slight bend in your knees as you lower the weight toward the floor.
  - Keep your back flat and engage your core as you return to a standing position.
  - **Tip** : Start with light weights and focus on maintaining proper form to avoid injury.

5. Panels

- **Targeted muscles** : trunk, shoulders, back.
- **How to do it** :
  - Start in a forearm plank position, with your elbows directly under your shoulders and your body in a straight line from head to heels.
  - Hold this position for as long as possible, engaging your core muscles and keeping your hips level.
  - **Tip** : Try to hold the plank position for 30 seconds to one minute, and gradually increase your time as you build strength.

4. CREATE A STRENGTH TRAINING ROUTINE

To create a balanced strength training routine, it's important to target all major muscle groups throughout the week. Here's an example of how to organize your strength training sessions.

Beginner Routine (2-3 Days a Week)

- **Day 1** : Lower Body
  - Squats (3 sets of 12 reps)
  - Lunges (3 sets of 12 reps each leg)
  - Glute Bridges (3 sets of 15 reps)
- **Day 2** : Upper Body
  - Push-ups (3 sets of 10 reps)
  - Dumbbell Rows (3 sets of 12 reps)
  - Shoulder presses (3 sets of 12 reps)
- **Day 3** : Full Body
  - Weight lifting (3 sets of 10 reps)
  - Planks (3 sets of 30 seconds)
  - Dumbbell curl exercise (3 sets of 12 reps)

Average routine (3-4 days a week)

- **Day 1** : Lower Body + Core
  - Squats, lunges, deadlifts, planks
- **Day 2** : Upper Body
  - Push-ups, shoulder presses, rows, and triceps dips
- **Day 3** : Full Body or HIIT
  - A combination of cardio and strength training.

CHAPTER EIGHT: FLEXIBILITY AND MOVEMENT

Flexibility and mobility are often overlooked aspects of fitness, yet they are essential to maintaining the health and function of the body. Flexibility refers to the range of motion around a joint, while mobility focuses on the joint's ability to move freely and efficiently. Together, they contribute to improved posture, reduced muscle stiffness, and a lower risk of injury. In this chapter, we'll highlight the importance of flexibility and mobility, the benefits they bring, and some basic stretching and mobility exercises to incorporate into your routine.

1. THE IMPORTANCE OF FLEXIBILITY AND MOBILITY

As we age, our muscles and joints tend to become stiffer, reducing flexibility and mobility. Lack of flexibility can lead to discomfort in everyday activities, while poor mobility can increase the risk of injury during exercise. Improving these areas of fitness can make movement easier, more efficient, and less painful.

Benefits of flexibility

- **Improved Range of Motion** : Flexible muscles allow for a greater range of motion in the joints, making it easier to perform everyday activities, such as bending, reaching, or twisting, without any discomfort.
- **Reduce the risk of injury** : Flexible muscles and tendons are less likely to be strained or torn during physical activity. Stretching helps prepare muscles for movement, reducing the risk of injuries such as muscle strains or joint sprains.
- **Improve posture** : Tight muscles, especially in the hips, shoulders, and back, can cause poor posture. Stretching and improving flexibility can help correct these imbalances and better support your posture over time.
- **Better muscle recovery** : Stretching after exercise can improve blood circulation to the muscles, which helps with recovery and reduces post-workout soreness.

Benefits of mobility

- **Joint Health** : Movement exercises help lubricate joints and keep them functioning optimally, reducing stiffness and discomfort.
- **Improves performance** : Movement allows you to make more efficient and powerful movements, whether you're lifting weights, running, or doing yoga. It also helps prevent compensatory movements that can lead to injury.
- **Balance and coordination** : Improving mobility enhances body awareness and balance, which is especially important for preventing falls and maintaining coordination as we age.

2. FLEXIBILITY VS. MOBILITY: UNDERSTANDING THE DIFFERENCE

Although flexibility and mobility are often used interchangeably, they are not the same thing. Understanding the difference between them will help you tailor your workouts to meet specific goals.

- **Flexibility** : Refers to the length and ability of a muscle to stretch. For example, being able to touch your toes is a sign of hamstring and lower back flexibility.
- **Movement** : Involves moving joints through a full range of motion with control. Movement involves strength and flexibility around the joint. For example, being able to squat deeply requires hip and ankle movement, along with strength in the legs and trunk.

Flexibility and mobility are both important, but they each serve different purposes. Flexibility exercises (such as static stretching) target muscles, while mobility exercises (such as dynamic stretching or yoga poses) focus on joints and the muscles around them.

3. BASIC FLEXIBILITY EXERCISES

Incorporating flexibility exercises into your daily routine can improve your overall range of motion, reduce muscle tension, and increase relaxation. Here are some key stretches that target major muscle groups and improve flexibility.

1. Hamstring muscle strain

- **Targeted muscles** : hamstrings, lower back.
- **How to do it** :

  1. Sit on the floor with your legs extended straight out in front of you.
  2. Bend at your hips and reach your arms forward toward your toes, keeping your back straight.
  3. Hold this position for 20-30 seconds, feeling the stretch in the back of your legs.

2. Quadriceps stretch

- **Targeted muscles** : quadriceps, hip muscles.
- **How to do it** :

  1. Stand straight and bend one knee, bringing your foot towards your glutes.
  2. Grab your ankle and gently pull it towards your body, feeling the stretch in the front of your thigh.
  3. Hold for 20-30 seconds, then switch legs.

3. Hip muscle tension

- **Targeted muscles** : hip muscles, quadriceps.
- **How to do it** :

  1. Start in a lunge position with your back knee on the floor and your front foot stationary.
  2. Move your hips forward until you feel a stretch in the front of your hip and thigh.
  3. Hold for 20-30 seconds, then switch legs.

4. Shoulder extension

- **Targeted muscles** : shoulders and upper back.
- **How to do it** :

  1. Extend one arm across your chest.

2. Use your opposite hand to gently pull the arm closer to your chest.
3. Hold for 20-30 seconds, then switch arms.

5. Butterfly exercise

- **Targeted muscles** : inner thighs and hips.
- **How to do it** :

1. Sit on the floor with the soles of your feet together and your knees bent out to the sides.
2. Hold your feet together and gently press your knees toward the floor.
3. Hold this position for 20-30 seconds, feeling the stretch in your inner thighs and hips.

Flexibility training tips:

- **Warm up first** : Always warm up before stretching. Stretching cold muscles can strain or injure them. A light warm-up (such as brisk walking or cycling) is ideal.
- **Breathe deeply** : While stretching, focus on taking slow, deep breaths. This helps relax your muscles and increase your range of motion.
- **Don't overstretch** : Stretching shouldn't be painful at all. Move into each stretch gently and stop when you feel a moderate stretch, avoiding any sharp or uncomfortable pain.

4. BASIC MOVEMENT EXERCISES

Mobility exercises are dynamic movements that improve range of motion and joint function. These exercises are especially beneficial for athletes and anyone looking to improve performance and reduce the risk of injury.

1. Cat and Cow Exercise (Spinal Movement)

- **How to do it :**

    1. Start on your hands and knees in a tabletop position.
    2. Arch your back (cat pose) by tucking your chin into your chest and rounding your spine.
    3. Then, reverse the movement by dropping your belly toward the floor and lifting your head (cow pose).
    4. Move between these positions for 30 seconds to improve spinal mobility.

2. Hip Circles (Hip Movement)

- **How to do it :**

    1. Stand with your feet shoulder-width apart and your hands on your hips.
    2. Slowly rotate your hips in a circular motion, moving clockwise and counterclockwise.
    3. Perform 10 circles in each direction to improve hip mobility.

3. Shoulder rolls (shoulder movement)

- **How to do it :**

    1. Stand or sit with your arms at your sides.
    2. Slowly move your shoulders forward in a circular motion, making large circles.
    3. After 10 reps, reverse the movement and move your shoulders back.

4. Thoracic rotation (upper back movement)

- **How to do it :**

   1. Sit or stand with your feet shoulder-width apart and your arms extended out to the sides.
   2. Rotate your torso to one side, keeping your hips stable and your arms extended.
   3. Return to center and then to the other side.
   4. Do 10-12 rotations on each side to improve upper back mobility.

5. Ankle Circles (Ankle Movement)

- **How to do it :**

   1. Sit or stand with one foot off the floor.
   2. Slowly rotate your ankle in a circular motion, making complete circles.
   3. Perform 10 circles in each direction, then switch feet.

Tips for movement training:

- **Be consistent** : Range-of-motion exercises can be done daily and are especially helpful when done before a workout. Consistency will help you improve your range of motion over time.
- **Focus on control** : Move slowly and with control during movement exercises. The goal is to increase joint flexibility while maintaining stability.
- **Use mobility tools** : Use foam rollers or massage balls to target tight areas and relieve muscle tension.

5. HOW TO INCORPORATE FLEXIBILITY AND MOBILITY INTO YOUR ROUTINE

Every fitness workout should include flexibility and mobility exercises, whether you're lifting weights, running or doing yoga. Here's how to incorporate them into your schedule.

Daily stretching exercises:

- **Morning Routine** : Start your day with a 5-10 minute stretching session to loosen up your muscles and prepare your body for movement.
- **Post-Workout** : Always include 5-10 minutes of static stretching at the end of your workout to help your muscles recover and improve flexibility.

Weekly movement exercises:

- **Pre-workout mobility exercises** : Perform dynamic mobility exercises, such as hip circles and arm swings, before exercise to increase joint range of motion and reduce the risk of injury.
- **Yoga or Pilates** : Incorporate yoga or Pilates into your weekly routine to improve flexibility, mobility, and balance. These practices combine static and dynamic stretches for a full-body workout.

Consistency is key:

The benefits of flexibility and mobility training come with consistent practice. Set aside time each day or week to work on improving these areas, and over time, you will notice a significant improvement in the quality of your movement and overall well-being.

CHAPTER 9: CARDIO EXERCISES FOR FAT LOSS AND IMPROVED HEART HEALTH

Cardiovascular exercise, or "cardiovascular exercise," is a staple of any fitness program, offering numerous benefits for both fat loss and heart health. Whether you're looking to lose weight, build endurance, or improve your heart's efficiency, cardiovascular exercise can help you achieve these goals. This chapter will explore the science behind cardiovascular exercise, discuss different types of cardiovascular exercise, and offer tips on how to incorporate it into your routine for maximum effectiveness.

1. WHAT IS CARDIOVASCULAR EXERCISE?

Cardiovascular exercise involves sustained physical activity that increases your heart rate and keeps it high for a long time. The main goal of cardiovascular exercise is to improve the efficiency of your cardiovascular system, which includes your heart, lungs, and blood vessels. During cardiovascular exercise, your heart pumps more blood, your lungs receive more oxygen, and your muscles use this oxygen for energy.

The main benefits of cardiovascular exercise:

- **Fat Loss** : Cardiovascular exercise is one of the most effective ways to burn calories and reduce body fat. It helps create a calorie deficit, which is essential for fat loss.
- **Heart Health** : Regular cardio exercise strengthens the heart muscle, improves blood circulation and reduces the risk of heart disease.
- **Increased stamina and endurance** : Cardio exercises enhance your body's ability to tolerate physical activity for extended periods, making everyday tasks easier.
- **Improve mental health** : Cardiovascular exercise releases endorphins, a natural mood booster in the body, which can help reduce stress, anxiety, and depression.
- **Better sleep** : Exercise can improve the quality of your sleep, making it easier to fall asleep and stay asleep throughout the night.

2. TYPES OF CARDIOVASCULAR EXERCISES

Cardiovascular exercise comes in many forms, from low-intensity activities like walking to high-intensity interval training (HIIT). The type of cardiovascular exercise you choose depends on your fitness goals, current fitness level, and personal preferences.

1. Steady-state cardio

- **What it is** : Steady-state cardiovascular exercise involves maintaining a steady, moderate pace for an extended period of time. This type of cardiovascular exercise keeps your heart rate steady without any sudden spikes.
- **Examples** : running, cycling, swimming, brisk walking, rowing.
- **Benefits** : Steady-state cardio is great for beginners and those looking to improve their endurance. It burns fat and calories efficiently and is easier on the joints than high-intensity cardio.
- **Duration** : Usually lasts between 30 to 60 minutes.

2. High-intensity interval training (HIIT)

- **What it is** : High-intensity interval training involves short periods of high-intensity exercise followed by short periods of rest or lower-intensity activity. This type of training raises your heart rate rapidly, followed by recovery periods.
- **Examples** : 30-second sprint followed by 1-minute walk, circuit training with exercises like burpees, jumping jacks, and mountain climbers.
- **Benefits** : HIIT workouts are extremely effective at burning fat and improving cardiovascular fitness in a short period of time. They also increase the "afterburn" effect, which means your body continues to burn calories even after your workout.
- **Duration** : Usually lasts for 20 to 30 minutes due to the high intensity of the exercise.

3. Low-impact cardio exercises

- **What it is** : Low-impact cardiovascular exercise that reduces stress on joints while still providing a cardiovascular challenge. These exercises are great for individuals recovering from injury or those who prefer gentler movements.
- **Examples** : walking, cycling, swimming, using an elliptical machine.
- **Benefits** : Low-impact cardio is ideal for people with joint problems, the elderly, or those new to exercise. It can be done for longer periods of time without causing strain or discomfort.
- **Duration** : Can be done for 30 to 60 minutes or more.

4. Dance-based cardio

- **What it is** : Dance-based cardio includes activities like Zumba, aerobics, or any exercise routine that involves rhythmic, dance-like movements.
- **Examples** : Zumba, aerobics, dance and fitness classes.
- **Benefits** : Dance-based cardio is fun, social, and engaging, making it easy to stick to a routine. It's a great way to burn calories while having fun.
- **Duration** : Usually lasts between 45 to 60 minutes.

5. Circuit training

- **What it is** : Circuit training combines strength training with cardio intervals. This type of exercise keeps your heart rate up while also building muscle.
- **Examples** : A combination of exercises such as push-ups, squats, kettlebell swings, and jumping jacks, performed in a circuit with minimal rest between exercises.
- **Benefits** : Circuit training is time-efficient and provides cardiovascular and strength benefits in one workout.
- **Duration** : Usually lasts 20 to 40 minutes, depending on the number of circuits.

3. CARDIO EXERCISES TO BURN FAT

Cardio is often associated with fat loss because it burns calories and helps create a calorie deficit, which is essential for shedding body fat. However, the type and duration of cardio, combined with a balanced diet, determines how effective it is in achieving your fat loss goals.

How Cardio Helps Burn Fat

When you exercise, your body uses glycogen (stored carbohydrates) and fat as a source of energy. During low- to moderate-intensity cardio, your body primarily burns fat for fuel. During high-intensity cardio, glycogen is used more for energy, but your overall calorie burn is higher, leading to fat loss over time.

Balancing cardio and strength training

Although cardiovascular exercise is effective in losing fat, it must be balanced with strength training to maintain muscle mass. Strength training boosts your metabolism and helps shape your body, ensuring that you don't lose muscle along with fat.

Best Cardio Exercises for Fat Loss

- **HIIT** : HIIT workouts are very effective for fat loss because they burn a large number of calories in a short period of time and create an "afterburn" effect, where your body continues to burn calories after your workout.
- **Steady-state cardiovascular exercise** : Long, moderate-intensity cardio sessions, such as brisk walking or jogging, are also effective for burning fat, especially when combined with a healthy diet.
- **Circuit Training** : This form of aerobic exercise combines fat burning with muscle building exercises, making it ideal for those looking to lose fat and build lean muscle at the same time.

4. CARDIOVASCULAR EXERCISES FOR HEART HEALTH

Cardiovascular exercise is essential for maintaining heart health and reducing the risk of heart disease. It strengthens the heart muscle, improves blood circulation, lowers blood pressure and helps control cholesterol levels.

How Cardio Exercise Helps Improve Heart Health

- **Strengthening the heart** : Like other muscles in the body, the heart gets stronger with exercise. A stronger heart pumps more blood with each beat, which improves circulation and reduces stress on the heart.
- **Lowering blood pressure** : Regular exercise helps lower systolic and diastolic blood pressure, reducing the risk of heart attacks and strokes.
- **Improve cholesterol levels** : Cardiovascular exercise increases levels of high-density lipoprotein (HDL), or "good" cholesterol, while lowering low-density lipoprotein (LDL), or "bad" cholesterol.
- **Reducing the risk of heart disease** : Cardiovascular exercise is one of the most effective ways to prevent heart disease by improving the efficiency of the cardiovascular system and maintaining a healthy weight.

Best Cardio Exercises for Heart Health

- **Walking** : A low-impact, moderate-intensity activity that can be done anywhere. Walking for 30 minutes a day at a brisk pace can significantly improve heart health.
- **Cycling** : Another low-impact exercise that strengthens the heart and improves cardiovascular endurance. It's also great for building lower body strength.
- **Swimming** : Swimming provides a full-body workout that is easy on the joints but very effective for heart health.
- **Running** : Running is a more intense form of cardio that greatly improves heart health and burns a lot of calories. However, it is higher impact, so it is important to use proper form and the right shoes to avoid injury.

5. HOW TO INCORPORATE CARDIO INTO YOUR ROUTINE

Cardiovascular exercise should be a regular part of your fitness routine, but the type and frequency of cardiovascular exercise depends on your fitness goals. Here are some tips for incorporating cardiovascular exercise into your schedule:

Beginner's Routine:

- **Frequency** : Start with 3-4 days of exercise per week.
- **Duration** : Aim for 20-30 minutes per session.
- **Type** : Choose low-impact exercises such as brisk walking, cycling, or swimming.

Average routine:

- **Frequency** : Increase to 4-5 days of exercise per week.
- **Duration** : Aim for 30-45 minutes per session.
- **Type** : Combine moderate-intensity exercises like running, dancing, or cycling with occasional HIIT sessions.

Advanced routine:

- **Frequency** : Incorporate aerobic exercise 5-6 days a week.
- **Duration** : 45-60 minutes per session.
- **Type** : Combines steady-state cardio, HIIT, and circuit training for maximum fat burning and endurance.

Track progress:

Use a fitness tracker or app to monitor your heart rate, calories burned, and distance covered during your cardio workouts. This will help you stay motivated and track your progress over time.

CHAPTER 10: YOGA AND PILATES TO STRENGTHEN THE CORE MUSCLES

Both yoga and Pilates are known for their ability to strengthen core muscles, improve posture, and enhance flexibility. While yoga focuses on the mind-body connection and breathing, Pilates emphasizes stability and controlled movement. Together, these practices offer a holistic approach to fitness that benefits both body and mind. In this chapter, we'll delve into how yoga and Pilates can help build core strength, improve balance, and reduce stress, along with key poses and exercises you can incorporate into your routine.

1. THE IMPORTANCE OF CORE STRENGTH

The core is often referred to as the body's "powerhouse." It includes the muscles of the abdomen, lower back, hips, and pelvis. A strong core is essential for maintaining good posture, supporting the spine, and providing stability during all types of physical activity. Whether you're lifting weights, running, or simply going about your daily activities, the core plays a vital role in every movement.

Benefits of core strength:

- **Improve Posture** : A strong core helps you maintain proper alignment, prevent hunching and reduce the risk of back pain.
- **Improves balance and stability** : Core strength contributes to better balance, making it easier to perform physical activities and reducing the likelihood of falls or injuries.
- **Injury prevention** : Strengthening your core muscles can help protect your spine and prevent injuries caused by poor posture or weak muscles.
- **Better Athletic Performance** : A strong core improves performance in sports and fitness activities by increasing control, strength and power.

Yoga and Pilates are two of the most effective exercises for building core abdominal muscles, as both focus on conscious, controlled movements that engage the deep abdominal muscles.

2. HOW YOGA HELPS BUILD CORE STRENGTH AND FLEXIBILITY

Yoga is an ancient practice that combines physical postures (asanas), breathing exercises (pranayama), and meditation to promote overall health. While yoga is often associated with flexibility and relaxation, it also offers significant benefits for strength and stability. Many yoga poses require balance and concentration, which naturally activates the body's muscles.

The main benefits of yoga:

- **Engaging the Deep Core Muscles** : Many yoga poses require activation of the transverse abdominis, obliques, and lower back, all of which contribute to core stability.
- **Improved flexibility and mobility** : Yoga improves flexibility by lengthening and stretching muscles, especially in the hips, spine, and shoulders. This increased flexibility helps prevent muscle imbalances that can lead to injury.
- **Mind-body connection** : Yoga helps you build awareness of how your body moves and functions, making you more aware of your posture and core engagement during daily activities.

Basic yoga poses to strengthen the core:

1. Plank Pose (Valakasana)

- **How to do it** :

    1. Start in a tabletop position with your wrists directly under your shoulders and your knees under your hips.
    2. Step your feet back one at a time, until you are in a straight-arm plank position with your body in a straight line from head to heels.
    3. Engage your core by pulling your belly button towards your spine, keeping your back flat.
    4. Hold this position for 20-30 seconds, gradually increasing the time as your strength improves.

2. Boat Pose (Navasana)

- **How to do it** :

    1. Sit on the floor with your legs extended in front of you.
    2. Lean back slightly, keeping your spine straight, then lift your legs so that your body forms a "V"

shape.

3. Extend your arms forward, parallel to the floor, and use your core muscles for balance.
4. Hold this position for 15-30 seconds, focusing on maintaining balance and engaging your abdominal muscles.

3. Downward Facing Dog (Adho Mukha Svanasana)

- **How to do it:**

  1. Start on your hands and knees in a tabletop position.
  2. Lift your hips up and back to form an inverted "V" shape, pressing your heels toward the floor and your hands firmly into the mat.
  3. Engage your core by pulling your belly button towards your spine and keeping your shoulders away from your ears.
  4. Hold this position for 30 seconds to 1 minute, breathing deeply to keep your core engaged.

4. Side Plank (Vasithasana)

- **How to do it:**

  1. Start in a high plank position with your shoulders over your wrists.
  2. Shift your weight to one hand and the outer edge of the same foot.
  3. Place your feet together and extend your opposite arm toward the ceiling.
  4. Engage your core to keep your body in a straight line and hold for 20-30 seconds on each side.

5. Bridge Pose (Setu Bandasana)

- **How to do it:**

  1. Lie on your back with your knees bent and your feet flat on the floor, hip-width apart.
  2. Press into your heels and lift your hips toward the ceiling while engaging your core and glutes.
  3. Hold this position for 20-30 seconds, then slowly

lower your hips down.

3. HOW PILATES EXERCISES IMPROVE CORE STRENGTH AND STABILITY

Pilates exercises, developed by Joseph Pilates in the early 20th century, focus on controlled movements and core stability. The practice emphasizes core strength, flexibility, and body alignment, making it an ideal complement to yoga or other forms of exercise. Pilates exercises are particularly effective at targeting the deep core muscles, including the transverse abdominis, pelvic floor, and lower back muscles.

The main benefits of Pilates:

- **Targeted Core Activation** : Pilates exercises are designed to isolate and activate the deep core muscles, which provide support and stability to the entire body.
- **Improve posture and alignment** : By strengthening the core and back muscles, Pilates exercises help correct posture and promote balanced spinal alignment.
- **Low Impact, High Benefits** : Pilates is low-impact, making it suitable for individuals of all fitness levels. It is gentle on the joints while providing a challenging core workout.

Basic Pilates exercises to strengthen the core muscles:

1. The hundred

- **How to do it :**
    - Lie on your back with your legs extended in the air at a 45-degree angle.
    - Lift your head, neck, and shoulders off the mat, and extend your arms out to the sides of your body.
    - Raise your arms up and down while inhaling for five counts and exhaling for five counts, to complete 100 pumps.
    - **Tip** : Keep your core muscles tight and your lower back pressed into the mat throughout the exercise.

2. Single leg stretch exercise

- **How to do it .**

    1. Lie on your back and bring your knees to your chest.
    2. Lift your head, neck, and shoulders off the mat, then extend one leg outward while keeping the other knee toward your chest.
    3. Switch legs, pulling the opposite knee toward your chest while extending the other leg.
    4. Continue alternating legs for 8-10 reps on each side, keeping your core engaged.

3. Roll up

- **How to do it** :
  - Lie on your back with your legs extended and your arms above your head.
  - Slowly roll your spine up, one vertebra at a time, and extend your arms toward your toes as you come to a sitting position.
  - Reverse the movement to return to the mat.
  - **Tip** : Engage your core muscles throughout the exercise and move slowly to control the roll up and down.

4. From board to pike

- **How to do it** :

  1. Start in a high plank position with your hands directly under your shoulders.
  2. Lift your hips toward the ceiling to form a spear pose (similar to downward facing dog in yoga).
  3. Lower your back into a plank position, keeping your core engaged the entire time.
  4. Repeat 10 to 12 times, focusing on controlled movement.

5. Scissors Kick

- **How to do it** :

  1. Lie on your back with your legs extended toward the ceiling.
  2. Lift your head, neck, and shoulders off the mat, then lower one leg toward the floor while keeping the other leg in the air.
  3. Alternate legs, simulating a scissors motion, keeping your core engaged.
  4. Perform 8-10 reps on each side.

4. BENEFITS OF COMBINING YOGA AND PILATES

Although yoga and Pilates are similar, they also have unique strengths that can complement each other when practiced together. Incorporating both yoga and Pilates into your routine can help you achieve a balanced body, combining flexibility, strength, and mental clarity.

Flexibility and strength:

- Yoga improves flexibility by stretching and lengthening muscles, while Pilates builds strength through controlled movements that focus on the core. Together, these two exercises help create a well-rounded fitness routine that balances movement and strength.

Posture and body stability:

- Pilates is particularly effective at improving posture by strengthening and stabilizing your core muscles, while yoga helps you maintain balance. Doing both exercises can improve your overall posture and reduce back pain.

Mindfulness and breathing:

- Yoga focuses on mindfulness and breathing, helping you develop a deeper connection with your body and mind. Pilates also involves controlled breathing, but its focus is more on precision and control of movement. Together, these exercises promote mental clarity and relaxation, reduce stress and improve overall health.

5. HOW TO INCORPORATE YOGA AND PILATES INTO YOUR ROUTINE

Both yoga and Pilates can be practiced separately or as part of a balanced fitness routine. Here's how to incorporate them into your weekly schedule:

Yoga routine:

- **Frequency** : Practice yoga 2-3 times a week to improve flexibility, balance, and mental clarity.
- **Duration** : Sessions can range from 30 to 60 minutes.
- **Type** : Focus on core-strengthening poses like plank, boat, and downward-facing dog, along with flexibility poses like forward bend and child's pose.

Pilates routine:

- **Frequency** : Incorporate Pilates exercises two to three times a week for core strength and stability.
- **Duration** : Pilates sessions usually last 30-45 minutes.
- **Type** : Focus on exercises like The Hundred, Roll-Up, and Scissor Kicks to strengthen your core and improve posture.

Compound routine:

- **Combine yoga and Pilates** : Some classes combine yoga and Pilates for a complete mind-body workout. You can alternate between the two or incorporate elements of each exercise into one session.

CHAPTER ELEVEN: DEBUNKING FITNESS MYTHS

When it comes to fitness, there is no shortage of advice, but not all of it is accurate. Fitness myths can create confusion, leading to ineffective workouts or even injury. In this chapter, we will debunk some of the most common fitness myths, ensuring you have the right information to achieve your goals efficiently and safely.

1. MYTH: "LIFTING WEIGHTS WILL MAKE YOU BULKY."

Fact: Strength training helps you build lean muscle.

One of the most common myths, especially among women, is the fear that lifting weights will make you gain huge muscles. The truth is that women generally do not have the hormonal makeup necessary to develop huge muscles like men. Testosterone, which is found in much higher levels in men, is the hormone responsible for muscle growth to a large extent.

For women, strength training results in increased muscle strength, improved tone, and a more sculpted appearance, not increased size. Even for men, achieving a massive physique requires specific training, a high-protein diet, and often years of consistent effort.

Benefits of weight lifting:

- **Definition of muscle gain** : Lifting weights helps create strong, toned muscles, giving you a more defined, sculpted appearance.
- **Boost your metabolism** : Muscle tissue burns more calories than fat, even at rest. Strength training increases your metabolism, which helps with fat loss and overall weight management.
- **Improve strength and function** : Strength training helps build functional strength that makes everyday tasks easier, from carrying groceries to lifting heavy objects.

2. MYTH: "YOU CAN REDUCE FAT IN SPECIFIC AREAS"

Fact: You can't target fat loss in specific areas.

Many people believe that exercising specific areas of the body—such as abs or thigh exercises—will reduce fat in those areas. This myth, known as "spot reduction," is unfortunately not how fat is lost. Fat is lost from the entire body, not just the areas you're exercising.

How does fat loss work:

When you exercise, your body uses energy from fat stores, but it doesn't select specific areas to pull fat from. For example, doing hundreds of sit-ups will tone your abdominal muscles, but it won't specifically reduce belly fat. Fat loss occurs through a combination of regular exercise (both cardio and strength training) and maintaining a calorie deficit—meaning you burn more calories than you consume.

What to do instead:

- **Focus on full-body exercises** : Combine cardio and strength training to burn fat from your entire body.
- **Be patient** : Fat loss happens gradually, and your body will decide where to lose fat first. Consistency is key.

3. MYTH: "MORE SWEAT MEANS A BETTER WORKOUT"

Fact: Sweat isn't always an indicator of a good workout.

Many people associate sweating with the effectiveness of a workout, but sweating isn't necessarily a sign of how hard you've worked. Sweating is your body's way of regulating temperature, and whether or not people sweat more or less varies depending on factors like genetics, humidity, and the type of exercise being performed.

For example, you might sweat a lot during hot yoga, but less during a strength training session, even though both exercises may be equally effective. The amount of sweat you sweat is not an indicator of calories burned or the intensity of your workout.

Better indicators of effective exercise:

- **Heart rate** : Monitoring your heart rate during exercise gives you a better understanding of the intensity of your workout. For cardiovascular health, try to keep your heart rate within 50-85% of your maximum heart rate (calculated as 220 minus your age).
- **Effort** : Pay attention to how hard you're working during your workout. If you're breathing harder, feeling a burn in your muscles, or pushing yourself harder, you're getting an effective workout, regardless of your sweat.

4. MYTH: "IF YOU'RE NOT SORE, YOU HAVEN'T TRAINED ENOUGH."

Fact: Muscle pain isn't always a sign of a good workout.

Many people believe that if they don't feel sore after a workout, they haven't worked out hard enough. However, muscle soreness — known as delayed-onset muscle soreness (DOMS) — isn't always an indicator of a successful workout. DOMS occurs when muscles are exposed to new or difficult stresses, causing microscopic damage. This leads to muscle soreness as the muscles repair and gain strength.

However, once your body adapts to certain exercises, you may feel less pain even as the exercise continues to be effective. Your muscles are still working, but they have become more efficient at handling stress, resulting in less pain after exercise.

What is more important than pain:

- **Progress** : Track your progress through measurable gains, such as lifting heavier weights, increasing your endurance, or improving your flexibility.
- **Consistency** : Focus on maintaining a regular exercise routine. You don't need to feel pain every time to know you're making progress.

5. MYTH: "CARDIO IS THE BEST WAY TO LOSE WEIGHT."

Fact: Combining strength training with cardio is most effective.

Although cardiovascular exercises, such as running, cycling, and swimming, are great for burning calories, they aren't necessarily the most effective way to lose fat in the long run. Relying solely on cardiovascular exercise for weight loss can lead to muscle loss, especially if you don't do strength training to maintain lean muscle mass.

Why Strength Training Is Important for Weight Loss:

- **Maintaining muscle mass** : Strength training helps maintain lean muscle mass while losing fat. Muscle tissue burns more calories at rest than fat, so maintaining muscle is key to boosting your metabolism.
- **Increases Calorie Burn** : After strength training, your body continues to burn calories as it repairs and rebuilds muscle tissue. This "afterburn effect" can last for several hours after your workout, making strength training an essential component of fat loss.
- **Improve Body Composition** : Strength training improves body composition by increasing muscle strength and reducing fat, giving you a leaner appearance.

Best approach:

- Combine **cardio and strength training** for optimal fat loss. Aim for a mix of aerobic exercise (like running or cycling) and strength training (like lifting weights or bodyweight exercises) throughout the week.

6. MYTH: "YOU HAVE TO EXERCISE DAILY TO SEE RESULTS."

Fact: Rest and recovery are as important as exercise.

Many people believe that exercising daily is essential to achieving fitness goals, but this can lead to burnout, injury, and overtraining. Rest and recovery are essential components of any fitness plan, allowing your muscles to repair, grow, and adapt to the stresses of exercise.

The importance of comfort:

- **Muscle Recovery** : Strength training causes microscopic tears in muscle fibers, which need time to recover and grow stronger. Overtraining without adequate rest can lead to fatigue, injury, and decreased performance.
- **Prevent Burnout** : Taking regular rest days helps prevent burnout and keeps you motivated to continue your fitness journey in the long run.
- **Mental and physical reset** : Rest days give your mind and body a chance to recharge, reducing the risk of mental fatigue and keeping your workouts fresh and effective.

Recommended recovery:

- **Active rest** : On rest days, consider doing light activities such as walking, stretching, or yoga to promote blood flow and help muscles recover.
- **Rest days** : Try to get at least one or two complete rest days per week, especially if you're doing strength training or intense cardiovascular exercise.

7. MYTH: "AB EXERCISES ARE THE BEST WAY TO GET TONED ABS."

Fact: Core strength comes from whole-body exercise and diet.

While crunches and sit-ups target your abdominal muscles, they aren't the most effective exercises for achieving a toned midsection. Crunches alone won't help you lose belly fat or show off defined abs. Combining full-body workouts, crunches, and a healthy diet is the key to building strong, defined abs.

What really works:

- **Full-body exercises** : Exercises like squats, deadlifts, and planks activate your core muscles along with other muscle groups, building overall strength and stability.
- **Core-specific exercises** : Incorporate exercises that target all areas of the core, such as planks, mountain climbers, and leg lifts.
- **Diet** : Abdominal muscles are primarily made in the kitchen. Reducing body fat through a balanced diet, portion control, and regular exercise will help show off the muscle mass in your abdominal area.

8. MYTH: "YOU SHOULD STRETCH BEFORE YOU EXERCISE."

Fact: Dynamic warm-ups are best before exercise.

For years, static stretching has been recommended as a warm-up before exercise. However, research has shown that stretching cold muscles before exercise can increase the risk of injury and reduce performance. Instead, dynamic warm-ups, which involve moving your muscles and joints through a full range of motion, are more effective at preparing your body for physical activity.

Examples of dynamic warm-up:

- **Leg Swing** : Swing your legs back and forth to relieve tension in your hips and hamstrings.
- **Arm Circles** : Rotate your arms in circular motions to warm up your shoulders.
- **Bodyweight Squats** : Perform squats to activate your legs, buttocks, and core.

Maintain static stretching after exercise when your muscles are warm, as it helps improve flexibility and promote recovery.

CHAPTER TWELVE: BEAUTY FOODS FOR HEALTHY SKIN AND HAIR

The adage "you are what you eat" is especially true when it comes to beauty. The foods we consume have a huge impact on the health and appearance of our skin, hair, and nails. While skincare products and treatments can enhance your outward appearance, true beauty starts from within. By nourishing your body with the right nutrients, you can promote healthy, radiant skin and strong, shiny hair. In this chapter, we'll explore some of the best beauty-boosting foods and how they contribute to your overall appearance.

1. ANTIOXIDANTS: FIGHT FREE RADICALS FOR A RADIANT COMPLEXION.

Antioxidants are compounds that protect the skin from damage caused by free radicals – unstable molecules that contribute to premature aging, wrinkles and dullness. Free radicals are caused by sun exposure, pollution and harmful chemicals, but antioxidants can neutralize them, prevent oxidative stress and promote healthy skin.

Top antioxidant-rich foods:

1. Berries (blueberries, strawberries, raspberries)

- **Why berries are good for your skin** : Berries are rich in antioxidants like vitamin C, which is essential for collagen production and maintaining skin elasticity. They also help fight skin inflammation and protect against environmental damage.
- **How to eat them** : Enjoy berries as a snack, add them to smoothies, or top your oatmeal with a handful for a beauty-boosting breakfast.

2. Dark chocolate (70% cocoa or higher)

- **Why it's good for your skin** : Dark chocolate contains flavonoids, which improve skin hydration and texture, protect against sun damage, and boost blood flow to the skin.
- **How to eat it** : Enjoy a small square of dark chocolate daily to satisfy your sweet tooth and promote healthy skin.

3. Green tea

- **Why it's good for your skin** : Green tea is rich in catechins, which help protect skin cells from UV damage, reduce redness, and improve hydration. It also has anti-inflammatory properties that can soothe irritated skin.
- **How to use** : Drink green tea throughout the day or apply chilled green tea bags to your skin to reduce puffiness and dark circles.

2. HEALTHY FATS: NOURISH YOUR SKIN AND HAIR FROM WITHIN

Healthy fats are essential to keeping your skin and hair moisturized and soft. Omega-3 fatty acids, in particular, help strengthen the skin barrier, reduce inflammation, and promote scalp health. A lack of healthy fats in your diet can lead to dry, flaky skin and brittle hair.

Best healthy foods rich in fat:

1. Avocado

- **Why it's good for your skin and hair** : Avocados are rich in healthy monounsaturated fats and vitamin E, both of which help keep skin soft, moisturized, and protected from oxidative stress. The fats in avocados also nourish the scalp, promoting shiny, healthy hair.
- **How to eat it** : Mash avocado on toast, add it to salads, or blend it into smoothies for a creamy texture and beauty benefits.

2. Fatty fish (salmon, mackerel, sardines)

- **Why it's good for your skin and hair** : Fatty fish is rich in omega-3 fatty acids, which help reduce inflammation, support skin hydration, and prevent acne. These healthy fats also promote hair growth and add shine.
- **How to eat it** : Try to eat fatty fish two to three times a week. You can also grill or bake salmon, or add sardines to salads for a dose of omega-3.

3. Nuts and seeds (walnuts, flax seeds, chia seeds)

- **Why they're good for your skin and hair** : Walnuts, flax seeds, and chia seeds are excellent sources of omega-3 fatty acids, antioxidants, and vitamins. These nutrients help fight inflammation, improve skin elasticity, and encourage hair growth.
- **How to eat it** : Sprinkle flax or chia seeds on yogurt or cereal, and enjoy a handful of walnuts as a snack.

3. VITAMINS AND MINERALS: ESSENTIAL ELEMENTS FOR HEALTHY SKIN AND HAIR

Certain vitamins and minerals are essential for maintaining healthy skin and hair. These micronutrients work at the cellular level to repair and regenerate tissue, keep skin supple, and promote strong, healthy hair.

Essential vitamins and minerals for beauty:

1. Vitamin C

- **Why it's good for skin and hair** : Vitamin C is essential for the formation of collagen, which keeps skin firm and youthful. It also lightens the skin and helps get rid of dark spots caused by sun damage. In addition, vitamin C strengthens hair and promotes its growth.
- **The best foods rich in vitamin C** : oranges, kiwi, strawberries, sweet peppers, and broccoli.
- **How to eat it** : Snack on citrus fruits, add bell peppers to your meals, and add broccoli to stir-fries.

2. Biotin (Vitamin B7)

- **Why it's good for hair** : Biotin is known for its role in promoting strong, healthy hair and preventing hair loss. It also supports healthy skin and nails.
- **The best foods rich in biotin** : eggs, almonds, sweet potatoes, spinach, and salmon.
- **How to eat it** : Include eggs in your breakfast, eat almonds as a snack, or roast sweet potatoes for a nutrient-rich side dish.

3. Zinc

- **Why it's good for your skin** : Zinc plays a key role in healing wounds, reducing inflammation, and keeping your skin acne-free. It also regulates the production of oils in your skin, preventing clogged pores and breakouts.
- **The best foods rich in zinc** : oysters, pumpkin seeds, chickpeas, and lean meats.
- **How to eat it** : Add pumpkin seeds to salads or yogurt, and add chickpeas to soups and stews to boost zinc.

4. Vitamin E

- **Why it's good for skin and hair** : Vitamin E is a powerful antioxidant that helps protect skin from environmental damage. It also improves skin hydration and elasticity, while promoting scalp health and preventing hair breakage.
- **The best foods that contain vitamin E** : almonds, sunflower seeds, spinach, and olive oil.
- **How to eat it** : Drizzle olive oil on salad, eat almonds as a snack, and sauté spinach with garlic for a nutritious side dish.

4. HYDRATION: WATER-RICH FOODS FOR GLOWING SKIN

Hydration is key to maintaining healthy skin and hair. When you're dehydrated, your skin can become dry, flaky, and prone to wrinkles. Drinking enough water is essential, but eating foods rich in water can also help keep your skin and hair hydrated from the inside out.

Best Hydrating Foods:

1. Option

- **Why cucumber is good for your skin** : Cucumber is made up of about 95% water, making it an excellent hydrating food. Cucumber also contains silica, a mineral that supports skin elasticity and hydration.
- **How to eat** : Add cucumber slices to salads, smoothies or infused water to boost your beauty.

2. Watermelon

- **Why it's good for skin** : Watermelon is hydrating and rich in vitamins A and C, both of which promote skin glow and prevent damage from free radicals.
- **How to eat it** : Enjoy watermelon as a snack, blend it into smoothies, or make a hydrating fruit salad with watermelon, mint, and lemon.

3. Leafy vegetables (spinach, cabbage, lettuce)

- **Why they're good for your skin** : Leafy greens are full of water and contain vital nutrients like vitamins A, C, and E, all of which promote healthy, youthful skin.
- **How to eat it** : Add spinach or kale to salads, smoothies, or stir-fries for a hydrating, nutrient-rich meal.

5. PROTEIN: THE BUILDING BLOCK
FOR HAIR GROWTH

Protein is essential for the formation of every cell in the body, including skin and hair. Hair is made primarily of a protein called keratin, so getting enough protein is crucial for hair growth, strength, and preventing breakage.

Best Protein-Rich Foods:

1. Eggs

- **Why it's good for hair** : Eggs are a rich source of high-quality protein and biotin, both of which promote hair growth and strengthen hair follicles.
- **How to eat it** : Start your day with scrambled eggs, an omelet, or hard-boiled eggs for a portable snack.

2. Lean meats (chicken, turkey, beef)

- **Why meat is good for hair** : Lean meat provides complete proteins that contain all the essential amino acids needed for hair growth. It also provides iron, which supports healthy blood flow to the scalp.
- **How to eat it** : Include lean meats such as grilled chicken or turkey in your meals to ensure you get enough protein to support hair growth.

3. Lentils and beans

- **Why they're good for hair** : Lentils and beans are excellent plant-based sources of protein, along with zinc and iron, which help promote hair growth and scalp health.
- **How to eat them** : Add lentils to soups, stews, or salads, and include beans in tacos, burritos, or as a side dish.

6. SUPERFOODS TO BOOST BEAUTY

Superfoods are nutrient-dense foods that provide a wide range of vitamins, minerals and antioxidants. Including these superfoods in your diet can greatly enhance your beauty, supporting glowing skin, strong hair and overall health.

Best Superfoods for Beauty:

1. Sweet potatoes

- **Why they're good for your skin** : Sweet potatoes are rich in beta-carotene, a precursor to vitamin A, which helps protect skin from sun damage and promotes a healthy glow.
- **How to eat them** : You can roast sweet potatoes as a side dish, or mash them for a nutrient-rich addition to your meals.

2. Greek yogurt

- **Why it's good for skin and hair** : Greek yogurt is high in protein, probiotics, and B vitamins, which help improve skin elasticity, boost collagen production, and support hair growth.
- **How to eat it** : Enjoy Greek yogurt with fresh fruit, honey or nuts for a nutrient-rich snack.

3. Pomegranate

- **Why it's good for skin** : Pomegranates are packed with antioxidants and vitamin C, which protect skin from environmental damage and promote youthful skin.
- **How to eat it** : Add pomegranate seeds to salads, yogurt, or smoothies for a refreshing and nutritious dose.

CHAPTER 13: CLEAN EATING AND MEAL PLANNING

Clean eating is more than just a diet, it's a lifestyle that focuses on whole, minimally processed foods that provide essential nutrients for optimal health, beauty, and fitness. By focusing on clean, nutrient-dense ingredients, you can provide your body with the vitamins and minerals it needs for glowing skin, strong hair, and peak physical performance. In this chapter, we'll explore the basics of clean eating, its benefits, and how to build a weekly meal plan that supports your beauty and fitness goals.

1. WHAT IS CLEAN EATING?

Clean eating is a way of choosing foods that are as close to their natural state as possible. It emphasizes eating whole, unprocessed foods and avoiding refined, artificial, and processed ingredients. Clean eating encourages you to pay attention to what you put into your body, and focus on nourishing yourself with real, whole foods rather than counting calories or following strict diets.

Basic principles of clean eating:

- **Eat whole foods** : Focus on fresh, unprocessed foods that are free of additives or preservatives, such as fruits, vegetables, whole grains, lean proteins, and healthy fats.
- **Avoid processed foods** : Limit or eliminate processed, packaged, or artificially added foods. This includes refined sugars, trans fats, artificial sweeteners, and pre-packaged snacks.
- **Choose nutrient-rich options** : Prioritize foods that are rich in nutrients, such as vitamins, minerals, fiber, and healthy fats. These foods nourish your body and provide it with energy for a long time.
- **Read labels** : Be aware of what's in the foods you buy by reading ingredient lists. Choose products with minimal ingredients, and avoid foods with added sugars, artificial flavors, or chemical additives.
- **Stay hydrated** : Drink plenty of water throughout the day and avoid sugary drinks, sodas, and excessive caffeine. Hydration is essential for healthy skin, hair, and overall vitality.

Clean eating is not about deprivation or strict rules, it's about making informed choices that support your health and well-being, while allowing for balance and pleasure at the same time.

2. BENEFITS OF HEALTHY EATING FOR BEAUTY AND FITNESS

Eating healthy is one of the most effective ways to enhance your natural beauty and improve your fitness levels. By eating whole, nutrient-rich foods, you provide your body with the tools it needs to grow from the inside out.

Beauty benefits:

- **Glowing Skin** : Eating clean reduces inflammation and promotes healthy skin by providing antioxidants, vitamins and healthy fats that protect skin from environmental damage and boost collagen production.
- **Stronger Hair and Nails** : Nutrient-rich foods like lean proteins, healthy fats, and vitamins A, C, and E help strengthen hair and nails, reduce brittleness, and promote growth.
- **Clearer skin** : Eating healthy helps you cut down on processed foods and refined sugars, which can contribute to acne and breakouts. Eating a whole-foods diet can help balance your hormones and keep your skin clear.

Benefits of fitness:

- **Increased Energy** : Clean, whole foods provide sustained energy throughout the day, improving your workout performance and boosting endurance. You won't suffer from the crashes that come with processed foods high in refined sugars.
- **Improve recovery** : Eating a diet rich in antioxidants, protein, and healthy fats helps muscles recover and reduces inflammation after intense workouts.
- **Better Body Composition** : Eating clean supports a balanced intake of macronutrients (proteins, fats, and carbohydrates), helping you build lean muscle and maintain a healthy body weight.
- **Stable blood sugar levels** : Whole foods, especially those high in fiber, help regulate blood sugar levels, prevent energy dips and keep your metabolism stable.

3. HOW TO BUILD A BALANCED MEAL PLAN

Creating a healthy meal plan doesn't have to be complicated. By focusing on a balance of macronutrients (protein, healthy fats, and complex carbohydrates) and incorporating a variety of whole foods, you can create nutritious meals that support your beauty and fitness goals.

Step 1: Prioritize nutrient-dense whole foods.

The foundation of your meal plan should be whole foods rich in essential nutrients. Try to include the following food groups in your meals:

- **Fruits and vegetables** : These fruits and vegetables contain vitamins, minerals, fiber, and antioxidants that promote healthy skin, hair, and overall well-being. Try to eat a variety of colorful fruits and vegetables to ensure you get a variety of nutrients.
- **Lean Proteins** : Protein is essential for muscle repair, hair growth, and skin health. You can eat protein sources such as chicken, turkey, fish, eggs, tofu, beans, and legumes.
- **Healthy fats** : Fats are essential for hormone production, brain function, and skin hydration. Eat healthy fats like avocados, olive oil, nuts, seeds, and fatty fish.
- **Whole grains** : Complex carbohydrates, such as quinoa, brown rice, oats, and whole wheat, provide sustained energy and are rich in fiber, which aids digestion and keeps skin healthy.
- **Hydration** : In addition to water, eat hydrating foods such as cucumber, watermelon, and leafy greens to help keep skin hydrated and flush out toxins.

Step 2: Plan your meals around macronutrients.

A balanced meal contains a mix of macronutrients - proteins, fats and carbohydrates. Each of the macronutrients plays a key role in fueling your body and promoting beauty and fitness.

- **Proteins** : Essential for muscle repair, growth, and overall tissue health. Make sure to include a source of lean protein at every meal.
- **Fats** : Healthy fats provide long-lasting energy, support brain function, and nourish your skin and hair. Include healthy fats in your meals, such as avocados, olive oil, or nuts.
- **Carbohydrates** : Choose complex carbohydrates that provide fiber and energy. Whole grains, sweet potatoes, and legumes are excellent choices that help you feel full and satisfied.

Step 3: Include snacks and hydration.

Healthy snacks and adequate hydration are essential components of healthy eating. Choose nutrient-rich snacks to keep your energy levels stable throughout the day.

- **Healthy snack ideas** :
  - A handful of almonds and a piece of fruit.
  - Greek yogurt with chia seeds and berries.
  - Vegetable sticks with hummus or guacamole.
- **Moisturizing** :
  - Drink water throughout the day, aiming for 8-10 glasses.
  - Herbal teas and water infused with fruits or herbs can add flavor and keep you hydrated without added sugar.

4. SAMPLE HEALTHY EATING MEAL PLAN

Here's a sample three-day clean eating meal plan to help you get started creating nutritious, balanced meals that support your beauty and fitness goals.

First day

- **Breakfast** :
    - Greek yogurt with a mix of berries, chia seeds and a little honey.
    - Green tea.
- **lunch** :
    - Grilled chicken salad with a variety of vegetables, avocado, cherry tomatoes, lemon and olive oil dressing.
    - A side of quinoa.
- **Snack** :
    - Apple slices with almond butter.
- **dinner** :
    - Baked salmon with roasted sweet potatoes and steamed broccoli.
    - A cup of water with lemon.

Day 2

- **Breakfast** :
    - Overnight oats with rolled oats, almond milk, flax seeds, and a handful of blueberries.
    - herbal tea.
- **lunch** :
    - Quinoa and black bean bowl with avocado, roasted veggies and a sprinkle of pumpkin seeds.
    - A side of mixed vegetables.
- **Snack** :
    - A handful of nuts and bananas.
- **dinner** :
    - Stir fried tofu with brown rice, sautéed spinach, and steamed carrots.
    - Water with cucumber slices.

Day 3

- **Breakfast** :
    - Scrambled eggs with spinach, mushrooms and a slice of whole grain toast.
    - Juice made from cabbage, cucumber, green apple and ginger.
- **lunch** :
    - Turkey and avocado wraps in whole wheat tortillas with a variety of veggies and carrot sticks.
    - Water with mint leaves.
- **Snack** :
    - Greek yogurt with 1 tablespoon sunflower seeds and berries.
- **dinner** :
    - Grilled shrimp with quinoa, steamed asparagus and a mix of mixed greens with

olive oil and balsamic vinegar.
- A cup of water.

5. TIPS FOR STICKING TO A HEALTHY DIET

Sticking to a healthy eating plan can be difficult, especially with busy schedules and temptations. Here are some tips to help you stay on track:

- **Meal Prep** : Preparing your meals ahead of time can help you avoid making unhealthy food choices when you're pressed for time. Cook in batches and store portions in the refrigerator or freezer.
- **Shop smart** : When grocery shopping, stick to the outside aisles where whole foods like fresh produce, meats, and dairy are located. Avoid processed and packaged foods in the middle aisles.
- **Read labels** : Pay attention to ingredient lists and choose products that contain minimal ingredients and no added sugars, preservatives or artificial flavors.
- **Allow for flexibility** : Healthy eating doesn't have to be strict. It's okay to indulge in snacks or convenience foods from time to time. The key is to make healthy choices most of the time and focus on balance, not perfection.
- **Stay hydrated** : Drink water regularly to keep your body hydrated and aid in digestion. Hydration plays an important role in maintaining clear skin and a healthy metabolism.

CHAPTER FOURTEEN: THE RELATIONSHIP BETWEEN MIND AND BODY IN BEAUTY AND FITNESS

In the pursuit of beauty and fitness, it's easy to focus only on the physical aspects—diet, exercise, and skincare. However, true health and beauty come from nurturing the relationship between your mind and body. The state of your mental and emotional health has a direct impact on how you look and feel. This chapter explores the powerful connection between mind and body, highlighting how managing stress, practicing mindfulness, and enhancing emotional well-being can elevate your beauty and fitness.

1. THE IMPACT OF MENTAL HEALTH ON PHYSICAL APPEARANCE

Our emotions, thoughts, and mental state affect the way we present ourselves physically. Stress, anxiety, and other negative feelings can manifest in a variety of ways—through breakouts, dull skin, hair loss, and even weight gain. Conversely, when we prioritize our mental health, we not only feel better, but we also radiate beauty from within.

How stress affects your skin and hair:

- **Pimples and Acne** : Stress increases the production of cortisol, a hormone that stimulates oil production in the skin. This excess oil can clog pores, leading to acne. Chronic stress also weakens the skin's barrier, making it more susceptible to irritation and inflammation.
- **Dull, dry skin** : High levels of stress deplete your skin of moisture, leaving it dry and lackluster. Stress also impairs your skin's ability to repair itself, which can make you look tired and aged.
- **Hair loss** : Stress can cause hair loss and thinning by pushing hair follicles into a resting phase, known as **telogen effluvium** , where they fall out more easily. This condition can last for several months, affecting the volume and health of your hair.
- **Weight gain or loss** : Stress can also affect weight by affecting your appetite and metabolism. Some people may overeat in response to stress, leading to weight gain, while others may lose their appetite, leading to unhealthy weight loss.

Positive effects on mental health:

- **Glowing Skin** : When you are emotionally balanced, your body produces fewer stress hormones, which promotes radiant skin. Being alert and relaxed also improves circulation, delivering oxygen and nutrients to the skin, creating a natural glow.
- **Healthy Hair** : Mental health supports the growth of strong, shiny hair. By managing stress and developing a positive mindset, you can reduce the risk of hair loss and promote a healthy scalp.
- **Better body composition** : When your mental health is under control, you're more likely to make healthier lifestyle choices, such as eating a balanced diet and getting a regular exercise routine. This, in turn, supports a healthy body weight and muscle strength

2. THE ROLE OF MINDFULNESS
IN BEAUTY AND FITNESS

Mindfulness is the practice of being fully present in the moment, without judgment. When applied to beauty and fitness, mindfulness can enhance your overall experience by helping you stay in tune with your body's needs and fostering a sense of self-appreciation. Mindfulness practices can improve how you approach skincare, eating habits, and exercise, creating more balanced and sustainable results.

Skin care with awareness:

Instead of rushing through your skincare routine, practice mindfulness by fully engaging with each step. Pay attention to the texture and smell of your products, and how they feel on your skin. Not only does this make your routine more enjoyable, it also helps you focus on what your skin really needs, whether it's extra hydration, exfoliation, or sensitive skin care.

- **Skin care benefits** :
    - Improves the effectiveness of products when applied intentionally.
    - Reduces stress by turning skincare into a relaxing self-care ritual.
    - It helps you identify changes in your skin and adjust your routine accordingly.

Mindful eating:

Mindful eating involves slowing down and paying attention to the sensory experience of eating, as well as the hunger and fullness signals your body sends. By being more present during meals, you're more likely to make healthier food choices, control portion sizes, and improve digestion.

- **Benefits of mindful eating** :
    - Helps you avoid overeating by recognizing when you are full.
    - Reduces stress and improves digestion by encouraging a calm, focused eating environment.
    - It enhances your appreciation for food, making healthy eating more enjoyable.

Conscious movement:

Whether you're doing yoga, running, or strength training, paying attention to your body's movements can improve the effectiveness and enjoyment of your workout. Focus on the feeling of your muscles as they contract, the flow of your breath, and the rhythm of your movements. This awareness helps prevent injury and ensures you're using proper form, while fostering a deeper connection to your body.

- **Benefits of conscious movement** :
    - Enhances exercise performance by improving focus and alignment.
    - Reduces the risk of injury by encouraging body awareness and proper form.
    - It increases enjoyment and helps you stay motivated to exercise regularly.

3. MEDITATION: A POWERFUL TOOL FOR REDUCING STRESS

Meditation is one of the most effective practices for managing stress, improving mental clarity, and promoting emotional health. Regular meditation helps regulate stress hormones like cortisol, which in turn supports clearer skin, healthier hair, and better overall health. Incorporating meditation into your daily routine can help reset your mind, improve your mood, and promote relaxation.

Benefits of meditation for beauty and fitness:

- **Reduces skin problems caused by stress** : By reducing stress levels, meditation helps reduce acne, irritation, and other skin conditions that are aggravated by stress.
- **BOOSTS MENTAL FOCUS AND MOTIVATION** : A clearer mind allows you to stay focused on your fitness goals and maintain a positive attitude toward healthy eating and exercise.
- **Promotes Better Sleep** : Meditation improves the quality of sleep, which is essential for skin repair, muscle recovery, and maintaining a youthful appearance.

Simple meditation techniques:

- **Breath awareness meditation** : Focus on your breath as it enters and exits your body. Breathe deeply and slowly, paying attention to each inhalation and exhalation. If your mind wanders, gently bring your focus back to your breath. Practice this for 5-10 minutes a day to reduce stress and improve focus.
- **Body Scan Meditation** : Close your eyes and mentally scan your body from head to toe, paying attention to any areas of tension or discomfort. Relax each area as you move through it, releasing physical and emotional tension.
- **Guided Meditation** : Use a meditation app or online resource to follow a guided meditation. This can be helpful for beginners and can focus on topics like relaxation, gratitude, or self-love.

4. STRESS MANAGEMENT FOR A HEALTHY MIND AND BODY

Managing stress is essential not only for your mental health but also for your physical appearance and fitness performance. Chronic stress negatively impacts every part of your body, from your skin and hair to your digestion and muscle recovery. Learning how to manage stress effectively can dramatically improve your beauty and fitness results.

Strategies for managing stress:

1. Physical activity:

- Exercising is one of the best ways to relieve stress. Physical activity increases the production of endorphins, a hormone that naturally improves mood, and lowers cortisol levels.
- Whether it's a vigorous run, a yoga session, or a muscle-strengthening workout, moving your body can help clear your mind, improve your mood, and promote better skin health by increasing circulation.

2. Deep breathing exercises:

- Deep breathing helps activate the parasympathetic nervous system, which helps the body relax and reduces the "fight or flight" response caused by stress.
- Practice deep breathing by slowly inhaling through your nose for four seconds, holding your breath for four seconds, and then exhaling through your mouth for four seconds. Repeat for 5 to 10 minutes to calm your mind.

3. Journaling:

- Writing down your thoughts and feelings can help you process emotions, relieve stress, and gain a better perspective on stressful situations.
- Try to set aside a few minutes each day to write about your experiences, challenges, and the things you're grateful for. Journaling can also help you track your progress on your fitness and beauty journey.

4. Adequate sleep:

- Sleep is a powerful tool for managing stress and supporting beauty and fitness. Lack of sleep increases cortisol levels, which can negatively impact your skin, hair, and energy levels.
- Make sure to get 7-9 hours of good sleep each night to allow your body and mind to fully recover. Create a calming bedtime routine, avoid screens before bed, and create a comfortable sleeping environment.

5. THE POWER OF POSITIVE THINKING AND SELF-LOVE

Your mindset plays a major role in how you perceive yourself and how you approach your beauty and fitness goals. A positive mindset encourages self-care, promotes emotional resilience, and leads to better physical outcomes. Practicing self-love and positive thinking can help you appreciate your body for what it can do, rather than focusing solely on how it looks.

How to develop a positive mindset:

- **Practice gratitude** : Start each day by listing a few things you're grateful for, whether it's your health, a recent accomplishment, or supportive relationships. This shifts your focus toward positivity and reduces stress.
- **Affirmations** : Use positive affirmations to boost self-love and self-confidence. Repeat phrases like "I am strong," "I am beautiful," or "I am capable" to remind yourself of your worth.
- **Have compassion for yourself** : Avoid harsh self-criticism and striving for perfection. Accept that progress takes time, and celebrate the small victories along the way. Treat yourself with the same kindness and understanding you would a friend.

CHAPTER 15: DEVELOPING A LONG-TERM FITNESS AND BEAUTY ROUTINE

Staying fit and healthy isn't just about short-term goals or quick fixes. True success lies in developing a consistent, sustainable routine that supports your physical and mental health. By adopting habits that become part of your daily life, you can achieve long-term results without the pressure of perfection or burnout. In this chapter, we'll explore how to create a flexible fitness and beauty routine, strategies for staying motivated, and the importance of evolving your goals as you go.

1. BUILD A SUSTAINABLE BEAUTY AND FITNESS ROUTINE.

Creating a lasting routine starts with finding the balance that works for you. A sustainable beauty and fitness routine should be manageable, enjoyable, and adaptable to life's ups and downs. The key is consistency, not perfection. Instead of aiming for extreme changes, focus on small, achievable steps that can be maintained over time.

Essential elements of a sustainable routine:

1. Consistency rather than intensity

- While high-intensity workouts and complex beauty routines may yield quick results, they're often difficult to sustain. It's best to prioritize consistency over intensity. Stick to daily habits, whether it's a 30-minute workout or a simple skincare routine, that fit easily into your schedule.
- **For example** : Instead of aiming for long, intense sessions in the gym five days a week, stick to shorter workouts, such as 20 to 30 minutes of cardio, strength training, or yoga, several times a week.

2. Flexibility and adaptability

- Life is unpredictable, and there will be times when you can't stick to your routine perfectly. The key is to allow flexibility in your plan. It's okay to adjust your schedule when needed, whether that's cutting back on exercise during a busy week or simplifying your skincare routine when time is tight.
- **For example** : If you miss a workout session, don't stress - just do it the next day or do a shorter version of your workout session at home.

3. Make it fun

- If you don't enjoy your daily routine, you're less likely to stick with it. Find activities and products that you truly enjoy and look forward to. Whether it's a fitness class that energizes you or a beauty ritual that relaxes you, make sure your daily routine enhances your life rather than feeling like a chore.
- **Example** : Try different types of exercise — dancing, swimming, strength training, or cycling — to find the one that makes you feel excited and motivated.

4. Set realistic goals.

- When creating your daily routine, set goals that are achievable, specific, measurable, and realistic. Avoid making drastic changes, and instead focus on gradual improvements. Realistic goals help you stay motivated and prevent burnout.
- **For example** : Instead of setting a goal to lose 10 pounds in one month, focus on adding three more workouts per week or increasing the amount of water you drink each day.

2. STRATEGIES FOR MAINTAINING MOTIVATION

Motivation can fluctuate, especially when it comes to long-term goals. It's normal to feel a little unmotivated at times, but having strategies in place can help you overcome stagnation and stick to your routine. Finding ways to stay inspired, accountable, and excited about your progress is essential to sustaining your beauty and fitness journey for the long term.

1. Track your progress

- Tracking your progress can boost your motivation by showing you how far you've come. Whether you measure your progress through fitness milestones (like lifting heavier weights or running faster) or by noticing improvements in your skin or hair, documenting your journey reminds you that your efforts are paying off.
- **How to track** : Use a fitness app, journal, or even photos to track physical changes, workouts, and skincare improvements over time.

2. Create small goals and rewards.

- Break your big goals down into smaller, achievable milestones and reward yourself when you reach them. This makes long-term goals seem more manageable and gives you something to look forward to.
- **Example** : If your goal is to exercise regularly, set a small goal of completing 10 exercises per month. Once you achieve that goal, reward yourself with something special, like a new workout outfit or a day at the spa.

3. Building a support system

- Surrounding yourself with supportive friends, family, or a fitness community can keep you accountable and motivated. Whether it's working out with a friend, joining a fitness class, or participating in an online beauty group, having people to share your journey with makes it more fun and keeps you on track.
- **For example** : Join a fitness challenge, take online yoga classes, or do a weekly check-in with a friend who shares similar beauty or fitness goals.

4. Embrace diversity and keep things new.

- Boredom is a common reason why people lose motivation in their beauty and fitness routines. To avoid this, mix things up by trying new exercises, skincare products, or beauty techniques. Variety keeps things interesting and prevents your routine from becoming monotonous.
- **For example** : Try a new skin care mask or switch up your workouts with different classes or outdoor activities like hiking or biking.

5. Focus on how you feel, not just how you look.

- While physical results like weight loss or clearer skin can be motivating, it's important to focus on how your routine makes you feel. Do you feel more energized, confident, or stressed? Changing your mindset to celebrate these internal improvements can help keep you motivated over time.
- **Example** : Keep a journal of how you feel after each workout or skincare session. Think

about the mental and emotional benefits, such as feeling more relaxed, clear-headed, or confident.

3. DEVELOP YOUR BEAUTY AND FITNESS GOALS OVER TIME.

As you progress on your beauty and fitness journey, your goals and needs will evolve. You may need to adjust what worked for you initially as you gain strength and experience or as your body's needs change. Flexibility is key to long-term success, and being open to new goals or routines will keep you engaged and motivated.

1. Re-evaluate your goals regularly.

- Every few months, take the time to reevaluate your fitness and beauty goals. Are you still aiming for the same results, or have your priorities changed? Adjusting your goals allows you to stay motivated and avoid stagnation.
- **Example** : If you were focused on losing weight and reached your goal, you might shift your focus to strength training, building muscle, or improving flexibility.

2. Change your routine to avoid stagnation.

- Doing the same exercises or using the same beauty products for too long can lead to a plateau, where you stop seeing progress. Changing your routine challenges your body and mind in new ways, helping you break through the plateau and continue to improve.
- **For example** : If you've been following the same strength training routine for several months, try adding new exercises, increasing the intensity, or incorporating different types of exercise such as Pilates or high-intensity interval training (HIIT).

3. Listen to your body's changing needs.

- As your body changes, so do its needs. You may need to adapt your routine to fit your current fitness level, age, or lifestyle. For example, as you age, you may need to focus more on flexibility, joint health, or recovery techniques like yoga or stretching.
- **For example** : If you find that high-impact exercises are becoming too hard on your joints, switch to low-impact exercises such as swimming, cycling, or walking while maintaining the intensity.

4. Celebrate long-term achievements.

- Long-term progress isn't just about hitting a certain number on the scale or getting clear skin. It's about building lifelong habits and maintaining your health and well-being. Celebrate long-term accomplishments, like sticking to your routine for six months or a year, and acknowledge the profound benefits you've experienced.
- **For example** : After completing a year of consistent exercise and skincare, reward yourself with something that supports your health and well-being, such as a weekend at the spa, a fitness trip, or an investment in new equipment or beauty tools.

4. INTEGRATING RECOVERY AND SELF-CARE

Recovery is just as important as your workout or beauty routine. Overtraining or neglecting rest can lead to fatigue, injury, or skin irritation. Incorporating recovery and self-care into your routine will help you sustain your efforts over the long term while keeping your mind and body in balance.

1. Prioritize rest days.

- Rest days allow your muscles to recover, repair, and grow stronger. Overtraining can lead to injury and burnout, so make sure to include at least one or two rest days a week in your fitness routine.
- **For example** : On rest days, focus on active recovery activities such as light stretching, yoga, or walking, which promote blood flow without stressing your body.

2. Integrate skin care to recover

- Just like your muscles need time to recover, your skin needs time to heal and regenerate. Use skincare products that support skin repair, such as serums with antioxidants, hydrating masks, or nutrient-rich oils.
- **Example** : Take a break from exfoliating or active ingredients (like retinol or acids) once a week to give your skin time to recover and repair.

3. Focus on sleep

- Good sleep is essential for muscle recovery, skin repair, and overall health. Aim for 7-9 hours of sleep each night to support your beauty and fitness goals. Sleep is the time when your body produces collagen, repairs damaged cells, and restores energy levels.
- **Example** : Create a bedtime routine that promotes restful sleep, such as turning off screens an hour before bed, practicing meditation, or using calming scents like lavender.

CHAPTER SIXTEEN: CONCLUSION AND FINAL ADVICE

Throughout this book, we explore the essential components of beauty and fitness—from skincare and nutrition to strength training and mindfulness. The ultimate goal is to create a balanced, sustainable approach to inner and outer wellness, allowing you to look and feel your best at any stage of life. In this final chapter, we'll conclude with key points and practical tips that will help you maintain your routine and continue to progress toward your beauty and fitness goals.

1. EMBRACE CONSISTENCY, NOT PERFECTION.

One of the most important lessons in both beauty and fitness is the value of consistency. Progress is achieved through small, consistent efforts over time, rather than drastic changes or perfection. Life will always present challenges, and there will be days when you can't stick to your routine perfectly. Instead of striving for perfection, focus on showing up consistently, whether that's by exercising for 20 minutes a few times a week or taking a few moments each day to pamper your skin.

Key tips:

- **Start small** : If you're just starting out, start with small, manageable steps, like adding one workout per week or focusing on hydration. Then gradually increase your routine over time.
- **Celebrate Progress** : Acknowledge the small victories you achieve along the way. Whether it's completing a workout or noticing clearer skin, these accomplishments will keep you motivated.
- **Allow for flexibility** : Life is unpredictable. If you miss a workout or have a snack, don't be hard on yourself. Just get back to your routine the next day.

2. PRIORITIZE SELF-CARE

Self-care is essential to maintaining balance and preventing burnout. Beauty and fitness aren't just about physical results; they're also about mental and emotional health. Incorporating self-care practices into your daily routine will help you recharge, reduce stress, and stay motivated in the long run.

Key tips:

- **Rest and Recovery** : Include rest days in your fitness routine and allow your skin to recover with moisturizing and soothing treatments. Overtraining and exfoliating can cause more harm than good.
- **Set boundaries** : Protect your time and energy by setting boundaries that allow you to focus on self-care. Whether it's turning off your phone at night or setting aside time to meditate, these practices will help you stay grounded.
- **Pamper yourself** : Every now and then, do activities that make you feel good, such as a day at the spa, a long bath, or a facial. Pampering yourself helps strengthen the connection between self-care and well-being.

3. MAINTAIN A BALANCE IN NUTRITION AND FITNESS.

A balanced approach to fitness and nutrition is essential for long-term health and beauty. Restrictive diets or intense workouts may yield short-term results but are difficult to maintain and can lead to burnout or injury. Focus on nourishing your body with a variety of whole foods and incorporating a mix of different types of physical activity.

Key tips:

- **Eat a variety of nutrient-dense foods** : Incorporate a wide variety of fruits, vegetables, lean proteins, whole grains, and healthy fats into your diet. This ensures that your body gets the essential nutrients it needs to thrive.
- **Find activities you enjoy** : Fitness should be something you look forward to, not a chore. Find physical activities you enjoy — whether it's yoga, dancing, swimming, or hiking — and make them part of your routine.
- **Listen to your body** : Your body will tell you when it needs rest, more food, or different types of movement. Listen to these signals and adjust your routine as needed.

4. DEVELOP A POSITIVE MINDSET

Your mindset profoundly impacts your beauty and fitness journey. A positive, growth-oriented mindset helps you stay motivated, overcome challenges, and appreciate the process. Instead of focusing solely on physical results, harness the emotional and mental benefits of taking care of yourself.

Key tips:

- **Practice gratitude** : Focus on the things you love about your body and the progress you've made. Gratitude shifts your thinking from what you lack to what you already have, helping you stay positive and motivated.
- **Affirmations** : Use positive affirmations to boost self-love and self-confidence. Phrases like "I am strong," "I am capable," and "I am beautiful" can empower you to continue making healthy choices.
- **Be kind to yourself** : Self-compassion is essential for long-term success. If you're having a bad day or don't achieve a goal, avoid being self-critical. Treat yourself with the same kindness you would a friend.

5. DEVELOP YOUR ROUTINE AS YOU GROW.

As your body changes and your life evolves, your beauty and fitness routine will change too. It's important to adjust your goals and methods as you age, progress, or take on new challenges. Being flexible in your routine allows you to stay engaged and continue to see results without feeling stagnant or bored.

Key tips:

- **Re-evaluate your goals regularly** : Every few months, take a moment to reflect on your progress and how you're feeling. Are you still working toward the same goals, or do you want to shift your focus to something new? This reflection will help keep your routine fresh and aligned with your current needs.
- **Try new activities** : Don't be afraid to explore new types of exercise, beauty products, or wellness practices. Trying new things keeps your routine exciting and allows you to discover new ways to care for your body.
- **Focus on longevity** : Instead of chasing short-term results, focus on building habits that will serve you throughout your life. Whether it's maintaining muscle strength, improving flexibility, or taking care of your skin, long-term beauty and fitness are all about feeling healthy and strong for years to come.

FINAL THOUGHTS: YOUR UNIQUE JOURNEY

Beauty and fitness are very individual things. What works for one person may not work for another, and your journey will be shaped by your own needs, preferences, and goals. The most important thing is to embrace your uniqueness, focus on what makes you feel good, and prioritize your well-being over societal pressures or trends.

Key points:

- **You are in control** : Your beauty and fitness journey is entirely in your hands. You have the power to make choices that benefit your body, mind, and spirit.
- **Health is more than just appearance** : While looking your best can boost your confidence, true beauty comes from feeling healthy, strong, and balanced from within. Focus on how you feel about your daily routine, not how you look.
- **Enjoy the Process** : The journey to better beauty and fitness is not a race, it's a lifelong process. Take time to appreciate your progress, enjoy your routine, and celebrate the small victories along the way.

ABOUT THE BOOK

Beauty & Fitness: A Holistic Approach to Wellness is your ultimate guide to achieving inner and outer beauty through sustainable wellness practices. This book combines science-backed fitness strategies, nutrition tips, skincare routines, and mental wellness techniques to help you look and feel your best. Whether you're just starting out on your journey or looking for new ways to elevate your self-care routine, this book covers everything from strength training and flexibility exercises to clean eating, mindfulness, and stress management.

This book is not just a fitness or beauty guide, it emphasizes the mind-body connection and the importance of balance, self-love, and consistency in your daily routine. By following the principles and techniques shared, you will be able to build a lifestyle that supports long-term wellness, empowering you to embrace your unique beauty and strength while nourishing your body and soul.

ABOUT THE AUTHOR

Veronica Balthazar

Veronica Balthazar has been a luminary in the world of cosmetology for over 40 years. Based in New York, USA, Veronica has dedicated her life to mastering the art and science of beauty. With a wealth of experience spanning several decades, she has honed her craft in some of the most prestigious salons and beauty institutes across the country. Her deep understanding of cosmetology and her passion for continuous learning have made her a highly sought-after professional in the industry. Veronica's expertise is not just limited to technical skills; she is also a mentor to many aspiring cosmetologists, sharing her knowledge through teaching, writing, and personal coaching. Through this ebook, Veronica Balthazar aims to share her lifetime of experience and insights, helping readers unlock the secrets of professional beauty techniques and succeed in their cosmetology careers.

BOOKS IN THIS SERIES

Unlocking The Secrets To Professional Beauty Techniques

"Unlocking the Secrets to Professional Beauty Techniques" is your ultimate guide to mastering the art of cosmetology. Whether you're a seasoned professional looking to enhance your skills or a newcomer eager to learn the trade, this book offers valuable insights and practical advice across a wide spectrum of beauty services. From advanced haircutting and styling techniques to skincare, makeup artistry, and nail care, this comprehensive guide covers it all. Packed with real-world case studies and expert tips, this ebook not only teaches you the "how-tos" of beauty but also the "whys," helping you understand the principles behind each technique to deliver stunning, customized results for every client. Dive in and discover how you can transform your passion for beauty into a thriving career!

Beauty And Fitness_ A Holistic Guide To Health And Wellness

Beauty & Fitness: A Holistic Approach to Wellness is your ultimate guide to achieving inner and outer beauty through sustainable wellness practices. This book combines science-backed fitness strategies, nutrition tips, skincare routines, and mental wellness techniques to help you look and feel your best. Whether you're just starting out on your journey or looking for new ways to elevate your self-care routine, this book covers everything from strength training and flexibility exercises to clean eating, mindfulness, and stress management.

This book is not just a fitness or beauty guide, it emphasizes the mind-body connection and the importance of balance, self-love, and consistency in your daily routine. By following the principles and techniques shared, you will be able to build a lifestyle that supports long-term wellness, empowering you to embrace your unique beauty and strength while nourishing your body and soul.